BEI GRIN MACHT SICH IHR WISSEN BEZAHLT

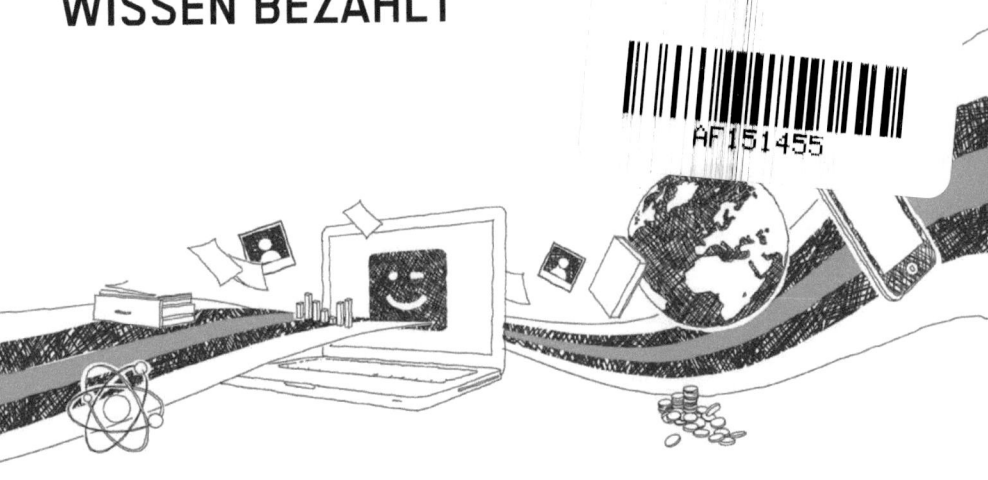

AF151455

- Wir veröffentlichen Ihre Hausarbeit, Bachelor- und Masterarbeit

- Ihr eigenes eBook und Buch - weltweit in allen wichtigen Shops

- Verdienen Sie an jedem Verkauf

Jetzt bei www.GRIN.com hochladen und kostenlos publizieren

GRIN

Ramesh Kumar Marya

Effects of Vitamin D Supplementation in Pregnancy and Lactation

An experimental Study

GRIN Verlag

Bibliografische Information der Deutschen Nationalbibliothek:

Die Deutsche Bibliothek verzeichnet diese Publikation in der Deutschen National-
bibliografie; detaillierte bibliografische Daten sind im Internet über http://dnb.d-
nb.de/ abrufbar.

Impressum:

Copyright © 2012 GRIN Verlag GmbH
Druck und Bindung: Books on Demand GmbH, Norderstedt Germany
ISBN: 978-3-656-47149-3

Dieses Buch bei GRIN:

http://www.grin.com/de/e-book/214738/effects-of-vitamin-d-supplementation-in-
pregnancy-and-lactation

GRIN - Your knowledge has value

Der GRIN Verlag publiziert seit 1998 wissenschaftliche Arbeiten von Studenten, Hochschullehrern und anderen Akademikern als eBook und gedrucktes Buch. Die Verlagswebsite www.grin.com ist die ideale Plattform zur Veröffentlichung von Hausarbeiten, Abschlussarbeiten, wissenschaftlichen Aufsätzen, Dissertationen und Fachbüchern.

Besuchen Sie uns im Internet:

http://www.grin.com/

http://www.facebook.com/grincom

http://www.twitter.com/grin_com

EFFECTS OF VITAMIN D SUPPLEMENTATION IN PREGNANCY AND LACTATION: EXPERIMENTAL STUDIES

by

R. K. Marya

CONTENTS

I. NTRODUCTION

II. REVIEW OF LITERATURE

A. HISTORICAL NOTE

B. VITAMIN D METABOLISM

C. MECHANISMS OF ACTION OF 1, 25 $(OH)_2$ D

D. BIOLOGICAL ACTIONS OF VITAMIN D

E. ROLE OF VITAMIN D IN PREGNANCY

F. ROLE OF VITAMIN D IN LACTATION

G. EFFECTS OF HYPOVITAMINOSIS D DURING PREGNANCY ON REPRODUCTIVE FUNCTION

III. MATERIALS & METHODS

IV. OBSERVATIONS

V. DISCUSSION

VI. SUMMARY

VII. BIBLIOGRAPHY

I. INTRODUCTION

Growth retardation is one of the well-known features of severe vitamin D deficiency in infants and young animals. It is generally assumed that skeletal growth retardation is due to sub-optimal concentrations of calcium and phosphorus in the extracellular fluids. The soft tissue growth retardation seen in severe vitamin D deficiency is attributed to anorexia induced by hypocalcemia. However, based upon their investigations in the rat, Steenbock and Herting (1955) proposed that vitamin D may have widespread effects on organic metabolism, of which growth is one manifestation. Recently nuclear receptor sites for 1,25, dihydroxy vitamin D3 (1,25 (OH)$_2$D3] have been reported in such diverse tissues as intestine, bone, skeletal muscle, cardiac muscle, mammary tissue, skin, testis, ovary, pancreas and parathyroid gland (Haddad and Birge, 1975; stumpf et al.,1979; Reichel et al., 1989). Even in the fetus, placenta, yolk sac , kidneys, bones and skin have nuclear receptor sites for 1,25 (OH)$_2$D3 (Haussler, 1986). These observations suggest that vitamin D, may have a more diverse physiological role than hitherto believed to be. Moreover, it has been observed that 1,25(OH)$_2$D3 promotes calcium binding protein synthesis in not only intestinal mucosa (a known target organ) but also in many of the tissues named above (Mayer et al., 1984; Clemens et al., 1985). Based on these reports, Haussler et al. (1985) have proposed that vitamin D may have a fundamental role in the regulation of cellular growth and differentiation.

It is generally accepted that daily administration of 100 IU of vitamin D is sufficient to prevent rickets in infants. However , clinical observations suggest that optimum growth may not occur when vitamin D intake of the infant is 100 IU per day. Stearns et al (1936) compared the length of infants on vitamin D supplements varying from 60-130 to 1800 IU per day. Optimum growth was shown by infants receiving 340-600 IU of vitamin D per day. Both the lower and higher doses decreased growth significantly. These findings were subsequently confirmed by many workers (Slyker et al .,1937; Jeans and Stearns, 1938; Greer et al., 1981).

Severe vitamin D deficiency in pregnant women is known since long to produce congenital rickets (Maxwell- et al.,1939; Liu et al.,1940; snapper, 1956). However the possible role of vitamin D in reproduction including intrauterine growth of the fetus has attracted attention only recently. In chicks, vitamin D seems to be essential for proper egg hatchability (Henry and Norman, 1978) and for normal embryo development (Sunde et al.,1978).

Halloran and De Luca (1980a) have reported decreased fertility, decreased litter size and greater incidence of neonatal deaths in vitamin D deficient female rats. Administration of toxic dose of vitamin D (20, 000 IU per day) was also found to impede fertilization, if given before mating or produce degeneration and resorption of the implanted blastocyst if given in early pregnancy (Nebel and Ornstein, 1966). Toxic doses of vitamin D in pregnant rats also produced growth retardation in the fetus (Ornoy et al 1968) as well as structural alteration in the placenta (Nebel &Ornoy, 1971).

All these experimental studies on the effects of vitamin D on reproductive function have been performed either on vitamin D deficient animals where the results are clouded by the concurrent maternal malnutrition because of anorexia or in pregnant rats on toxic doses of vitamin D. Effect of administration of vitamin D in moderately high but non-toxic doses in pregnancy has not been studied. The apparent benefits of such a therapy on intrauterine and neonatal growth have been demonstrated in a few clinical studies by the author (Marya et al., 1981a ; Marya et al, 1981B) and others (Brooke et al, 1980; Maxwell et al., 1981). Studied by the author were conducted in Hindu women of Haryana, who in non-pregnant state, do not show any evidence of overt or occult vitamin D deficiency (Marya et al, 1981b). Administration of 600,000 units of vitamin D, in 7th and 8th months of pregnancy led to birth of infants with significantly greater birth weight and increase in certain other anthropometric measurements such as length, head circumference and skinfold thickness (Marya et al, 1981b). Administration of 1200 IU of vitamin D, per day, throughout the third trimester also improved the fetal birth weight but to a lesser extent (Marya et al., 1981a). Brooke et al. (1980) administered 1000 IU of vitamin D, per day to Asian immigrants in the U.K. during the third trimester of pregnancy and observed a significant decrease in the incidence of low birth weight babies. Although, there was no significant difference between the mean birth weight in the supplemented and non- supplemented groups but a follow up study revealed significantly greater weight and height of babies from the supplemented group at the age of 9 months and 12 months, even though neither the mothers nor the babies received any vitamin D supplements postnatal (Brooke et al., 1981) . The clinical studies suggest that administration of moderately high doses of vitamin D during pregnancy not only improves the intrauterine growth of the fetus but also continues to confer the beneficial effect on the growth of the baby during the first year of

4

life . However community nutritional studies are somewhat handicapped in that even when the subjects are taken from the same socio-economic strata of the society, the environmental and nutritional conditions cannot be rigidly controlled. These difficulties assume greater importance in the studies on vitamin D where subtle differences in the solar exposure, cutaneous pigmentation and manner of dress may produce important effects on the cutaneous production of vitamin D. Hence confirmation of the results obtained in human subjects by experimental studies in the rat was considered imperative. This study was designed to elucidate the effects of vitamin D supplementation during pregnancy on the skeletal and soft tissue growth in the rat pups.

II. REVIEW OF LITERATURE

A. HISTORICAL NOTE

Like most of the vitamins, the discovery of vitamin D was a consequence of the knowledge of its deficiency disorders. The first clinical description of rickets appeared in 1650 (Olson & De Luca, 1973) after the widespread appearance of rickets in northern Europe due to industrialization. The incidence of rickets reached serious proportions with the development of urbanized industrial population. Smoky skies coupled with relatively indoor life necessitated by this environment drastically reduced the solar exposure of the people, thereby curtailing the chief source of vitamin D. Cod-liver oil was recognized as a therapeutic measure for curing rickets in 1811 (Olson & De Luca, 1973). By the beginning of 20th century, the relation between dietary deficiency and many diseases such as beriberi and scurvy was demonstrated and the term vitamin was introduced by Funk in 1912 . In a series of publications, Mellenby (1918 a, 1918 b, 1919) demonstrated that rickets is a deficiency disease and it could be cured by cod-liver oil- or butter fat but attributed the cure to "fat soluble A." Huldscginsky in, 1920, provided the experimental proof of the curative effects of U.V. radiation on rickets (Olson & De Luca, 1973). In 1925, McCollum had the honor of naming the fourth discovered vitamin as vitamin D (McCollem et al, 1925). In 1924, Steenbock showed that phytosterol and ergosterol became rich in vitamin D after U.V. radiation (Steenbock, 1924; Steenbock & Black, 1925). Subsequently, vitamin D was crystallized from irradiated ergosterol and the compound was named calciferol (Askew et al, 1930; Windaus, 1932). In 1935, Windaus et al. determined the chemical structure of calciferol, and 7- dehydrochlesterol was shown to be a provitamin D. After this,

5

except for   official adoption of the name vitamin D_2, for   ergocalciferol   and vitamin D_3, for cholecalciferol (Patterson, 1952), the research activity   on vitamin D almost came to stand still. Only in late sixties, the role of the liver   and the kidney in vitamin D metabolism was elucidated. Since then, there has been a spurt of research activity on vitamin D and every year hundreds of papers appear in literature on various aspects of vitamin D metabolism.

B.   VITAMIN D METABOLISM

(i)   Cutaneous Production of Vitamin D

Diet is a very poor source of vitamin D. Vitamin D does not occur in vegetable kingdom. In non-vegetarian diet, egg and fish liver oil are the only important sources of vitamin D. Cow's milk is a poor source. However, cutaneous synthesis of vitamin is an important source of vitamin D. Most of the vitamin D synthesis occurs in the actively growing layers of the epidermis (strata spongiosum and basale) by exposure to   sunlight(Holick et al., 1980). Radiation energies between 290 and 320 nm are most effective (McLaughlin et al., 1982). 7-dehydro-cholesterol present in the epidermis acts as a provitamin D. Ultraviolet radiation produces a cleavage of B ring thereby forming previtamin D, (9,10 -secosteroid). Previtamin D undergoes a temperature dependent isomerization to form vitamin D_3 (also called cholecalciferol), taking 2-3 days for completion of the process . The unique thermally regulated synthesis of vitamin D_3 ensures a gradual release of the vitamin from the epidermis into circulation. This concept is confirmed by the observation that subjects exposed to whole body U.V. radiation have a significant increase in the circulating concentrations of vitamin D_3, about 6-9 hours after the exposure that reaches a peak 24-48 hours after the exposure, before gradually returning to baseline by 7 days (Adam et al., 1982). Once vitamin D is formed,   vitamin D-binding protein in the dermal capillary circulation   helps to   translocate   the vitamin from   blood-less epidermal tissue   into circulation.

Melanin pigment present in the epidermis interferes with the synthesis of vitamin D by absorbing U.V. radiation. The view of Loomis (1967) that skin pigmentation is evolved for the control of vitamin D synthesis in the skin is supported by excessive cutaneous melanin seen in populations exposed to greater U.V. radiation. Moreover, it has been observed that when surgically excised skins from Blacks and Caucasians were exposed to solar radiation, greater amount of vitamin D was produced in the latter (Holick et al., 1981). However, now it

6

is clear that melanin is only one of the many factors that regulate photosynthesis of vitamin D in the skin. Cutaneous production of vitamin D seems to be under an autoregulatory control. Excessive exposure of even Caucasian skin to sunlight does not cause vitamin D intoxication. Continuous exposure to UV radiation depletes cutaneous provitamin D, but does not increase production of previtamin D. Holick et al. (1981) have reported the effect of exposure of skin for different durations to sunlight. During the first 10-15 minutes of exposure, approximately 15% of provitamin D changed to previtamin D. After one hour of exposure, 40 % provitamin D was depleted but only 15 % increase in previtamin D was observed. The remaining 25% of photolyzed provitamin D was accounted for by the presence of inactive isomers, tachysterol and lumisterol (Fig. 1). Further solar exposure depleted the stores of provitamin D in the epidermis, but the concentration of previtamin D_3 or vitamin D_3 did not increase. Vitamin D_3 being heat-sensitive, may also be photodegraded to 5,6-trans-vitamin D_3 and suprasterol (Web et al, 1986).

Because of the complex mechanism of vitamin D_3 production in the epidermis, the amount of solar exposure required for providing vitamin D adequate for the body's requirements varies in different individuals and under different conditions. The photosynthesis of vitamin D_3 depends upon (i) the surface area of the skin exposed to sunlight, (ii) the time of the day of exposure (UV radiation is most intense between 11 AM and 2 PM) , (iii) the amount of melanin pigment present in the epidermis, (iv) latitude (UV radiation is most intense at the equator), (v) season (in winter less UV radiation reaches the surface of the earth, (vi) Environmental pollution such as smoke, fog and dust prevents UV radiation from reaching the earth. However, prolonged exposure to sunlight does not necessarily mean greater production of vitamin D since as mentioned earlier, solar radiation can isomerize previtamin D_3 to inactive, isomers, tachysterol and lumisterol as well as produce photodegradation of vitamin D_3 (Holick, 1986).

Vitamin D-binding protein has no affinity for tachysterol or lumisterol and hence translocation of these isomers into circulation does not occur. These products are sloughed off during natural turnover of skin. Patients with uremia seem to be unable to produce vitamin D in the skin. It is believed that one or more substances present in the skin of a patient with chronic renal failure act like melanin and absorb UV radiation (Holick, 1986)).

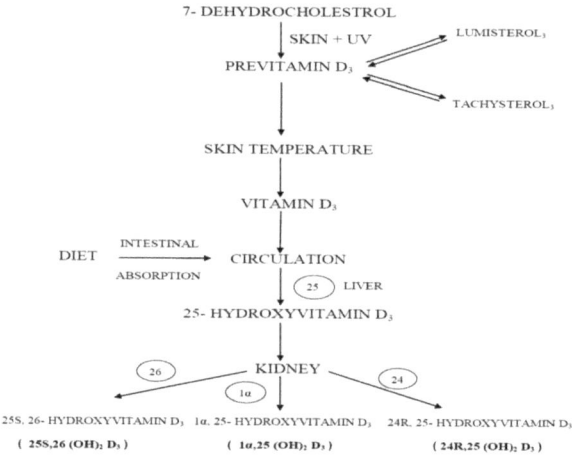

Fig.1. Vitamin D metabolism.

(ii)   Hepatic Metabolism of vitamin D

Vitamin D_3, synthesized in the skin, enters the circulation bound to vitamin D-binding protein. Dietary vitamin D_2 or D_3 enters the circulation through lymphatic system. Subsequently, both vitamins D_2 and D_3 are metabolized similarly.

In the liver, vitamin D is metabolized by vitamin D-25-hydroxylase to form 25-hydroxyvitamin D [25(OH) D] (now also known as calcidiol). The enzyme is located in the mitochondrial and microsomal fractions of the hepatocytes (Ponchon & DeLuca 1969; De Luca, 1984). Although there are few reports of the presence of extrahepatic vitamin D-25-hydroxylase in the chick and the rat (Tucker et al., 1973; Olson et al., 1976), the liver seems to be the only site of 25 (OH) D synthesis in humans. The reserve capacity of vitamin D-25-hydroxylase in the liver is substantial. Severe parenchymal damage is required to lower the level of plasma 25(OH) D (Long et al., 1976). The enzyme vitamin D-25-hydroxylase does not seem to be tightly regulated since circulating levels of 25(OH) D vary with the amount of dietary intake of vitamin D or with the degree of solar exposure (Holick et al., 1986). Decreased plasma 25(OH) D levels are observed in patients with nephrotic syndrome having proteinuria greater than 4g/day, due to renal loss of vitamin D tagged to vitamin D-binding protein (Pietrek & Kokot, 197).

(iii)   Renal Metabolism of Vitamin D

As early as 1833, Lucas recognized the association between chronic renal disease and bony lesions resembling rickets. Observations of similarity in bony lesions in patients of nutritional rickets and those with chronic renal failure, led Liu and Chu (1943) to propose that uremia interferes with the action of vitamin D. It was only in 1970 that Fraser& Kodicek demonstrated the intimate relation between the kidney and vitamin D metabolism. These workers demonstrated that homogenates of chick kidney could metabolize 25(OH) D to a biological active metabolite. It was also shown that physiological concentrations of 25(OH) D could not stimulate intestinal calcium transport in anephric rat (Boyle et al., 1972). Fraser & Kodicek (1970) identified the active metabolite as 1, 25-dihydroxycholecalficerol [1,25 $(OH)_2$ D_3] (now also known as calcitriol). The renal 25 (OH)-1- alpha-hydroxylase is located in the proximal convoluted tubules (Suda &Kurokova, 1983) . It is now accepted that 1, 25-dihydroxy metabolites of vitamin D_2 or D_3 are the biologically active forms of vitamin D_2 and D_3 respectively. These metabolites are 10 times more active than vitamin D_2 or D_3 in healing rickets or stimulating intestinal calcium absorption (De Luca, 1984).

The activity of renal 25-OH-1-alpha hydroxylase appears to be tightly regulated since plasma 1, 25 (OH) 2 D_3 concentration remains constant over a wide range of substrate 25 (OH) D_3. Parathormone (PTH) seems to play a crucial role in the synthesis of calcitriol since it was found that hypocalcemic vitamin D deficient rats could metabolize calcidiol to calcitriol more effectively than normocalcemic vitamin D replete rats (Boyle et al., 1971). But, when vitamin D- deficient hypocalcemic rats were thyroparathyroidectomized, the difference was lost (Garabedian et al., 1972). However, according to Holick et al. (1986), PTH may not be absolutely essential for the synthesis of 1, 25 $(OH)_2$ D, since patients with hypoparathyroidism often have low-normal concentrations of calcitriol. Under certain physiological conditions, factors other than PTH may regulate 1, 25 $(OH)_2$ D synthesis. In pregnanc and lactation, growth hormone, estrogens and prolactin seem to enhance renal production of 1,25 $(OH)_2$ D directly or indirectly (Baksi &Kenny, 1977; Boass et al., 1977) .

(iv)   Alternate Renal Metabolic Pathways for 25 (OH) D

When vitamin D nutrition and circulating plasma concentrations of calcium and phosphorus are normal, 25 (OH) D is metabolized into a variety of products (Fig. 1), by hydroxylation at C 24, 25 and 26 to form 1,25 $(OH)_2$ D, 24,25 $(OH)_2$ D and 25,26 $(OH)_2$ D (Holick et al., 1986). The plasma concentrations of each of 24, 25 $(OH)_2$ D and 25,26 $(OH)_2$D are 50-100 times the concentration of 1,25 $(OH)_2$ D. The metabolites other than 1, 25 $(OH)_2$ D have no biological activity. Production of 25 (OH) D is uncontrolled. Its plasma concentrations vary directly with the dietary intake/ cutaneous production of vitamin D. When plasma concentration of 1, 25 $(OH)_2D$ is adequate, remaining 25(OH) D is converted to 24,25 $(OH)_2$ D or 25,26 $(OH)_2$ D. Renal 25 (OH)-1-alpha-hydroxylase converts two inert metabolites mentioned above to 1,24,25 trihydroxy cholecalciferol [1,24,25 $(OH)_3$ D] and 1,25,26 trihydroxy cholecalciferol [1,25,26 $(OH)_3D$]. The trihydroxy metabolites again have no biological activity (De Luca, 1984).

(v)   Extrarenal Metabolism of 25(OH)D

Initially, kidney was believed to be the only site of 1, 25 $(OH)_2$ D synthesis. Twenty-four hours after injection of ^{3}H- 25(OH)D, ^{3}H-1,25 $(OH)_2$ D could be detected in the blood and tissues of vitamin D deficient rats but not in vitamin D deficient rats that had undergone bilateral nephrectomy before receiving radioactive 25 (OH) D (Gray et al., 1971). Later it was discovered that bilateral nephrectomy reduced, but did not abolish the conversion of 25(OH) D to 1, 25 $(OH)_2$ D (Weisman et al., 1978 b). In vitro studies have confirmed that placenta is the one of the sites for 1, 25 $(OH)_2$ D synthesis in pregnancy (Whitsett et al., 1981). In addition, in vitro, a wide variety of cultured cells from normal human bone, and osteosarcoma have a capacity to convert 25 (OH) D to 1, 25 $(OH)_2$ D (Turner et al., 1980; Howard et al., 1981; Howard et al, 1982). These observations also help to explain why hypercalcemia occurs in some patients of sarcoidosis, tuberculosis, silicosis, Hodgkin's disease and non-Hodgkin lymphoma. Such patients have been shown to have elevated plasma levels of 1, 25 $(OH)_2$ D (Gkonon et al., 1984; Breslau et al., 1984; Davies et al., 1985). To date, 25-OH-1-α-hydroxylase has been reported in many cells and tissues including prostate, breast, colon, lung, pancreatic β cells, monocytes, and parathyroid cells. However, the extrarenally produced 1, 25(OH)$_2$D primarily serves as an autocrine/paracrine factor with cell-specific functions [(Fig. 2) (Dusso et al., 2005)].

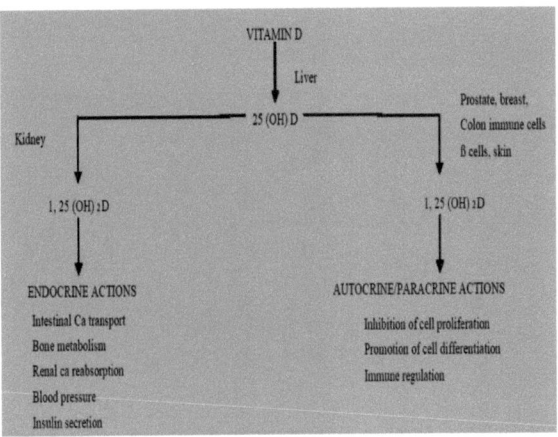

Fig.2. Renal and extrarenal production of 1,25-dihydroxyvitamin D. [After Dusso et al (2005)[.

C.   MECHANISMS OF ACTION OF 1, 25 (OH)$_2$ D

Vitamin D receptor (VDR) was discovered in 1968 (Haussler et al., 1968). In 1980s, VDR was found to be widely distributed in different tissues of the body such as gonads, stomach, epidermis, pituitary gland, pancreas, breast, parathyroid gland, thymus, cardiac muscle, skeletal muscle, placenta etc. (Stumpf et al., 1979; Mayer et al., 1984). Initially no physiologic significance was attached to such reports; only intestine, bone and kidney continued to be recognized as the target tissues of 1, 25 (25)$_2$ D. Subsequently, reports indicated calcium-binding protein synthesis in many of these tissues, including brain (Mayer et al., 1984). In vitro, 1, 25 (OH)$_2$ D was found to inhibit proliferation of human fibroblast cells and keratinocytes, increase TSH synthesis, inhibit PTH synthesis (Amento et al., 1984; Smith et al., 1986).

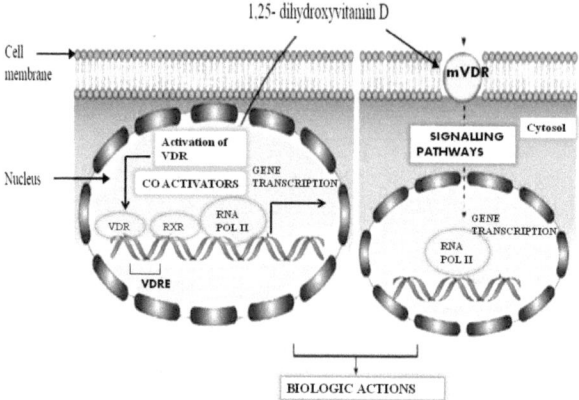

Fig. 3. Mechanism of genomic (left) and non-genomic (right) actions of vitamin D_3. (Adapted from Sergio et al., 2003).

(i)   **VDR and transcription regulation**

The genomic action of 1, 25(OH)$_2$ D$_3$ is well described. Most of the pleiotropic and long-term actions of 1, 25(OH)$_2$ D$_3$ are mediated through genomic actions. 1, 25(OH)$_2$D$_3$, in concert with vitamin D binding protein (DBP), is transported to the nucleus, where it binds to the vitamin D receptor (VDR). The VDR then complexes with retinoid X receptor (RXR), forming a heterodimer, which then binds the vitamin D-responsive element (VDRE) located in the promoter region of the gene. This association recruits either co-activators or co-suppressor molecules (depending on the tissue type). This triple complex then binds to the transcription machinery (Sergio et al., 2003 ;Fig. 3) .

(ii)   **Non-Genomic action of 1,25 (OH) D**

A variety of hormones, those serve as ligands for nuclear hormone receptors, also exert biological actions that do not require gene regulation. They seem to act through cell membrane receptor rather than nuclear receptors. 1, 25 (OH) $_2$ D$_3$ has been shown to have rapid effects in selected cells through membrane receptors. The proposed mechanism of non-genomic action of 1, 25 (OH)$_2$ D$_3$ is shown in Fig. 3.

D. BIOLOGICAL ACTIONS OF VITAMIN D

(i) Classical actions

The classical actions of vitamin D on the intestine, bone and kidney are concerned with calcium homeostasis.

(a) Intestine.

In the enterocytes of the small intestine, the genomic action of 1,25 $(OH)_2$ D_3 results in greater production of not only calcium binding protein, calbindin, but also alkaline phosphatase and a brush border protein (Mayer et al., 1984; Wasserman et al., 1984, Bickle & Munson, 1985).The net result is greater absorption of dietary calcium and phosphates. The mechanisms by which 1, 25$(OH)_2$ D_3 regulates transcellular calcium transport are best understood in the intestine. Here 1, 25$(OH)_2D_3$ stimulates calcium entry across the brush border membrane into the cell, transport of calcium through the cell, and removal of calcium from the cell at the basolateral membrane. Entry at the brush border membrane occurs down a steep electrochemical gradient. The molecular mechanism of 1, 25 $(OH)_2$ D_3 as a stimulator of intestinal phosphate absorption remains unknown, despite many efforts by the investigators (Jones et al., 1998), but a cytosolic calcium binding protein calbindin-D9K seems to be involved (Anderson et al 1998).

(b) Bone

Bone and muscle accumulate about 60% of injected dose of vitamin D (De Luca, 1976). Though gross skeletal abnormalities have been observed in vitamin D deficient animals, no direct effect of 1, 25 $(OH)_2$ D_3 on the process of ossification has been observed. 1, 25 $(OH)_2$ D_3 does not seem to be essential for ossification of bone. When plasma calcium and phosphate levels were maintained at normal range in vitamin D deficient rats by dietary manipulation, the skeletal histology was found to be normal (Holtrop et al., 1986). However, in cultured rat osteosarcoma cells, 1, 25 $(OH)_2$ D_3 stimulates the synthesis of osteocalcin , the bone derived protein, in a dose dependent manner (Price, 1984). In patients with postmenopausal osteoporosis, 1, 25 $(OH)_2$ D_3 administration has been shown to increase circulating osteocalcin levels (Zerwekh et al., 1985).

Mobilization of calcium from the bone is another well-known function of vitamin D, especially when administered in pharmacologic doses. At physiologic concentrations, 1, 25 $(OH)_2$ D_3 acts in concert with parathormone to stimulate osteoclastic activity (Garabedian et al., 1974). At pharmacologic concentrations, it was found to stimulate osteoclastic activity by inducing stem cells to differentiate into osteoclast cells (Haussler, 1986). Exposure to human peripheral monocytes that possess receptors for 1, 25 $(OH)_2$ D_3 results in their differentiation into multinucleated giant cells capable of mobilizing calcium from bone chips (Gray & Cohen, 1985).

(c) Kidneys

The most important endocrine effect of 1, $25(OH)_2D_3$ in the kidney is a tight control of its own homeostasis through simultaneous suppression of 1-α-hydroxylase and stimulation of 24-hydroxylase.

In the kidneys, 1, 25 $(OH)_2$ D increases reabsorption of calcium in the distal tubules through a cytosolic transport protein calbindin-D28K (Anderson et al., 1998). However, 1, $25(OH)_2$ D_3 involvement in the renal handling of calcium and phosphate continues to be controversial due to the simultaneous effects of 1, $25(OH)_2D_3$ on plasma PTH and on intestinal calcium and phosphate absorption, which affect the filter load of both ions .

(ii) Non-classic actions of vitamin D

1. Role of Vitamin D Hormone in the Parathyroid Gland

Perhaps the most well-established non-classic function of 1, $25(OH)_2$ D_3 is in the parathyroid gland. Specific localization of 1, $25(OH)_2$ D_3 in the parathyroid gland (Stumpf et al., 1979) and the presence of VDR (Henry & Newman, 1975) strongly suggested that $1,25(OH)_2$ D_3 may have a direct action through its receptor in the parathyroid glands. Moreover, PTH secretion by isolated parathyroid glands or cells could be suppressed by the direct administration of 1, $25(OH)_2$ D_3 (De Luca, 1976). Likewise, the vitamin D appears to be involved with the development of both primary and secondary hyperparathyroidism (Laundry et al., 2011). The specific mechanism by which vitamin D interacts with the parathyroid gland to bring about observed effects is not yet fully understood. But, these observations have implication on prospects of possible medical treatment of hyperparathyroidism (Hellman et al.,1999).

2. Role of Vitamin D Hormone in Skin

Hosomi et al. (1978) provided evidence for the first time that 1, 25(OH)$_2$ D$_3$ induces keratinocyte differentiation.. Exactly how important this differentiation effect of 1, 25(OH)$_2$ D$_3$ is in vivo is difficult to assess. Certainly, vitamin D-deficient animals do not have a problem with keratinocyte differentiation. Thus hyperproliferation of the keratinocyte and failure to differentiate is not found in vitamin D-deficient animals (De Luca, 1971). The differentiation of the keratinocyte is associated with an inhibition of proliferation. This inhibition of proliferation has been utilized in the treatment of hyperproliferative diseases of skin as, for example, psoriasis. Both 1, 25(OH)$_2$ D$_3$ and analogs can be used as a significant therapy against psoriasis with as many as 70% patients responding to this treatment (Parez et al., 1986). However, exactly how 1, 25-(OH)$_2$ D$_3$ induces differentiation of the keratinocyte and inhibits proliferation remains to be investigated. It has been proposed that the keratinocyte functions in a paracrine fashion in which 1, 25 (OH)$_2$ D$_3$ is produced by the keratinocyte itself to stimulate differentiation of the keratinocyte (Bickle et al., 1986).

3. Role of Vitamin D in the Immune System

The presence of the VDR in activated T lymphocytes was reported by Provvedine et al. (1987). These results suggested a role for 1, 25-(OH)$_2$ D$_3$ in the immune system, but the role is just now beginning to be defined. VDR have been reported in thymus, a repository of immature lymphocytes, as well. Vitamin D deficiency markedly reduces the ability of mouse to develop delayed hypersensitivity reaction (Young et al., 1983). These results suggest that T-helper cell lymphocyte is vitamin D responsive, but both immunostimulation and immunosuppression can be found in in vivo conditions. Currently, there is no evidence that B-lymphocyte-mediated immunity is influenced by 1, 25 (OH)2 D$_3$ (Jones et al., 1998).

The most dramatic results obtained to date in the immune system are those found in experimental autoimmune encephalomyelitis (EAE) that can be induced in mice. Administration of 1, 25 (OH)$_2$ D$_3$ suppressed the development of the disease in experimental animals(Fig 4) (Cantora et al., 1996). Current results strongly suggest that 1, 25 (OH)$_2$ D$_3$ or its analogues function by stimulation TH-2 T-helper cells to produce transforming growth factor-β1 and IL-4.

Of some interest is the idea that immunomodulation action of vitamin D might be useful in the management of transplant rejection (Jones et al., 1998). The possible use of vitamin D in the treatment of autoimmune diseases such as diabetes mellitus, rheumatoid arthritis is being investigated.

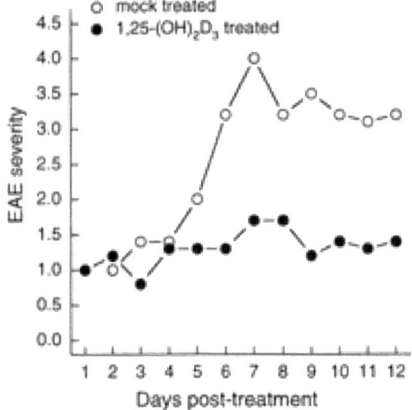

Fig. 4. Effect of administration of 1,25 (OH) 2 D_3 on the development of induced experimental autoimmune encephalitis in rats (After Cantorna et al., 1996)).

4. Role of vitamin D in Insulin Secretion.

The presence of a VDR in the cells of islets of Langerhans is now well accepted, but it is unclear as to what, if any, role vitamin D plays in the functioning of the islet cells. Initial results revealed that vitamin D-deficient rats were unable to respond to a glucose challenge by secreting appropriate amounts of insulin, which could be corrected by the administration of 1, $25(OH)_2 D_3$ (Cherotow et al., 1983). Other studies suggested that the effect of 1, 25 $(OH)_2 D_3$ was mediated by the action of vitamin D in raising plasma calcium concentration (Cherotow et al., 1986). Moreover, onset of experimental diabetes can be delayed by administration of 1, 25 $(OH)_2 D_3$ (Methian et al., 1992). Thus, a role of vitamin D on islet insulin release is most likely; either direct or indirectly through its effect on plasma calcium concentrations. Therefore, the relationship between vitamin D and diabetes is certainly worthy of further investigations.

5. Role of Vitamin D in Reproduction

Initially, during the course of producing vitamin D-deficient rats, came the observation that female reproduction is markedly diminished in vitamin D deficiency (Halloran & De Luca, 1980). An 80 % reduction in fertility was found and could not be corrected by correcting the hypocalcemia (Kwiecinski et al., 1989 a). This defect, therefore, is quite clearly one related to an absence of the vitamin D molecule. The infertility brought about by vitamin D deficiency in the female rat can be easily corrected by the administration of 1, 25-$(OH)_2D_3$ (Kwiecinski et al., 1989 b)). All such reports suggested that the ovary is a target of vitamin D action. More over the observations that ovarian cells contain VDR (Dokos et al., 1983) and 1, 25$(OH)_2$ D_3 accumulates in the ovarian cells (Stumpf et al., 1979) lends further support to the view.

In the case of male reproduction, vitamin D deficiency also reduces the effectiveness of the male (Kwiesinki et al., 1989). A significant reduction found in sperm count in vitamin D rats (Sood et al., 1992) could be reversed by vitamin D repletion (Sood et al., 1995). However, the diminished male fertility can also be corrected by merely providing additional calcium, raising plasma calcium concentration which in turn restores fertility (Kwiecinski et al 1989). In chicks, vitamin D seems to be essential for proper egg hatchability (Henry et al., 1978) and for normal embryo development (Sunde et al., 1978).

Severe vitamin D deficiency in human pregnancy is known since long to produce congenital rickets (Maxwell et al., 1939; Liu et al., 1940). The apparent benefits of vitamin D supplementation on intrauterine and neonatal growth of the fetus were initially demonstrated in Asian women by Brooke et al (1980) and by Marya and his colleagues (Marya et al., 1981; Marya et al 1984; Puri et al., 1989). Brooke et al. administered 1000 IU of vitamin D, per day to Asian immigrants in the U.K. during the third trimester of pregnancy and observed a significant decrease in the incidence of low birth weight babies. Although, there was no significant difference between the mean birth weight in the supplemented and non-supplemented groups but a follow up study revealed significantly greater weight and height of babies from the supplemented group at the age of 9 months and 12 months, even though neither the mothers nor the babies received any vitamin D supplements postnatal (Brooke et al., 1980). Studies by Marya and his colleagues (Marya et al., 1981; Marya et al 1984; Puri et al., 1989) were conducted in Hindu women of Haryana (India). Administration of 600,000 units of vitamin D, in 7th and 8th months of pregnancy led to birth of infants with significantly greater birth weight and increase in certain other anthropometric measurements such as length, head circumference and skinfold thickness . Administration of 1200 IU. of vitamin D, per day, throughout the third trimester also improved the fetal birth weight but to a lesser extent . The clinical studies suggest that administration of moderately high doses of vitamin D during pregnancy not only improves the intrauterine growth of the fetus but continues to confer the beneficial effect on the growth of the baby during the first year of life also.

The clinical and experimental studies led to a large number of studies on the effects of vitamin D supplementation during pregnancy on maternal and fetal outcomes. The rationality of such studies was the reports that women all over the world suffered from vitamin D deficiency during pregnancy (Dawood et al 2007; Sachan et al., 2005). Maternal vitamin D deficiency has been found to affect postnatal head and linear growth (Brunvand et al., 1996). Hollis et al. (2011) conducted a double blind trial on the possible benefits of vitamin D supplementation during pregnancy. It was concluded that vitamin D supplementation of 4000 IU/d for pregnant women is safe and most effective in achieving sufficiency in all women and their neonates regardless of race, whereas the currently suggested requirement is comparatively ineffective at achieving adequate circulating 25(OH)D concentrations, especially in African Americans.

De-Regil et al. (2012) conducted a Cochrane review of six randomized controlled trials in 1023 women. The results showed that the provision of vitamin D supplements during pregnancy improves the women's vitamin D levels, as measured by 25-hydroxyvitamin D levels, at term. However, the clinical significance of this finding is yet to be determined as there is no evidence that vitamin D supplementation prevents pre-eclampsia, gestational diabetes or impaired glucose tolerance. Data from three trials involving 463 women show a trend for women who receive vitamin D supplementation during pregnancy to less frequently have a baby with a birth weight below 2500 grams than those women receiving no treatment or placebo, although the statistical significance was border line. The number of trials and outcomes reported are too limited, and in general are of low quality, to draw conclusions on the usefulness and safety of this intervention as a part of routine antenatal care. Further rigorous randomized trials are required to evaluate the role of vitamin D supplementation in pregnancy (De Regil et al, 2012).

E.   ROLE OF VITAMIN D IN PREGNANCY

The study of vitamin D metabolism in pregnancy and lactation was prompted by the observations of osteomalacia in pregnant and lactating women in India and China (Maxwell and Miles, 1925; Ford et al. 1973). The requirement of the fetus for calcium during gestation and of the neonate during lactation puts considerable demand on the mother. Now, it is being realized that even Caucasian women tend to go into biochemical osteomalacia during pregnancy and lactation and need to be supplemented with vitamin D (Dawood and Wagner, 2007, Sachan et al., 2005;Watney and Rudd, 1974) .

(I)   Intestinal Calcium Absorption in Pregnancy

Greater calcium demands of the body during pregnancy and lactation can be met with by increasing the dietary calcium intake, or by increasing efficiency of intestinal calcium absorption mechanism or decreasing calcium losses in the urine. In rats as well as humans, increased appetite for food has been observed in pregnancy (Cripps and Williams, 1975, Toverud & Boass, 1979). But in women residing in developing countries, financial constraints limit the actual increase in intake of food. Obviously, increased efficiency of intestinal calcium absorption remains the chief mechanism of increasing availability of calcium to the mother. A marked increase in the efficiency intestinal calcium absorption in later months of pregnancy has been observed in humans (Heaney &Skillman, 1971) and sheep (Braithwaite et al. , 1970). It has been attributed to vitamin D as well as some other factors. Halloran et al. (1980 b) estimated intestinal calcium transport ratio (serosal Ca^{++}/ mucosal Ca^{++} ratio) in vitamin D-replete and vitamin D-deficient pregnant rats. The ratio was 6.0 in vitamin D-replete pregnant rats as compared to 3.0 in vitamin D-replete non-pregnant control rats. Surprisingly, the ratio was 3.5 in vitamin D-deficient pregnant rats as compared to 2.0 in vitamin D-deficient non-pregnant rats. In rats on a fixed dietary intake of vitamin D, the plasma concentrations of 25 (OH) D and 24, 25 $(OH)_2$ D decreased while that of 1,25 $(OH)_2$ D_3 and PTH increased during later days of pregnancy (Reitz et al., 1977; Halloran et al.,1979; Pitkin et al., 1979;Bouillon and De Moor, 1973). Such studies are cited to explain PTH-mediated increase in synthesis of 1, 25 $(OH)2$ D_3 during pregnancy leading to increased efficiency of intestinal calcium absorption. However, some workers have failed to observe increased plasma concentration of PTH during pregnancy (Wieland et al., 1980; Whitehead et al., 1981; Gillette et al., 1982). It has been suggested that during pregnancy, increased plasma levels of growth hormone, prolactin and placental lactogen stimulate 25 (OH) 1-alpha-hydroxylase activity in the kidney (Tanaka et al., 1976; Spanos et al., 1976; Baksi & Kenny, 1977; Baksi et al., 1978; Tanaka et al., 1978). Prolactin has been shown to increase intestinal calcium absorption not only in vitamin D-replete but also vitamin D –deficient animals (Mainoya, 1975 a, b; Pahuja and Deluca, 1981. The mechanism by which prolactin increases intestinal calcium is not exactly clear. Possibly, the effect of prolactin on calcium transport is mediated through intestinal mucosal hypertrophy. Prolactin is a tropic hormone for mammary glands. Similar action in the intestinal mucosa is quite likely (Harding & Cairnie, 1975; Maionoya, 1978). In pregnancy an increase in villus height, absorptive cell number and tissue weight has been reported (Cripps & Williams, 1975; Burdett & Ruk, 1979).

Renal conservation of calcium is another mechanism which may be utilized by the body for improving the availability of calcium to the fetus. However, due to increased GFR in later months of pregnancy, the excretion of many urinary constituents such as amino acids, glucose and calcium increases (Howarth et al., 1977; Marya et al., 1987; Maikranz et al., 1989;). Calcium conservation during pregnancy may be observed in in those with vitamin D-deficiency when the affected women tend to develop hypocalciuria (Marya et al., 1987). An association between hypocalciuria and pregnancy-induced hypertension has also been reported (Donovan et al., 2009).

(II)   Bone Metabolism in Pregnancy

The effect of pregnancy on bone metabolism is not entirely clear. It has been suggested that minerals accumulate in the bone during pregnancy in anticipation of calcium demands during lactation (Denzie et al, 1955; Heaney & Skillman, 1971). In vitamin D-deficient rat, there is roughly 25% increase in femoral bone mineral content by the end of pregnancy. In vitamin D-replete rat, however no change in mineral content could be demonstrated during pregnancy (Halloran % DeLuca, 1980 C). Many studies have suggested that in the rat under normal dietary conditions of vitamin D, calcium and phosphate intake, there is no change in bone mineral content during pregnancy. Under such conditions, the calcium requirements of the fetus and neonate are met with by increased intestinal calcium absorption (Naismith, 1966; Miller et al., 1982). Under conditions of dietary restriction of calcium, bone mineral is sacrificed to support fetal demands (Rasmussen, 1977 a, 1977 b).   Many workers have investigated the changes in bone mineral content in human pregnancy but results remain inconclusive (Gambaccini et al. 1995; Yamaga et al., 1996).

(III) Placental Calcium Transport

To meet the fetal demand, calcium is actively pumped across the placenta (Twardock & Austin, 1970). This view is supported by the observation of 1-2 mg% higher serum calcium level in fetus than in mother (Watney & Rudd, 1974). In the later months of pregnancy, increased rate of calcium transport in placenta is accompanied by appearance of calcium-binding protein in placenta. This protein has properties similar to those of intestinal calcium – binding protein associated with vitamin D induced transport of calcium in the intestine (Bruns et al.,1978: Dolorme et al., 1978). Thus, vitamin D may have a role in improving placental calcium transport. However, the amount of calcium transferred to the fetus during pregnancy in vitamin D-deficient female rats is slightly greater than that transferred in vitamin D-replete female. This observation suggests that the active transport of calcium across the placenta may not be dependent on vitamin D alone (Halloran &DeLuca, 1981). It seems, parathyroid hormone related peptide (PTHrP) is also involved in placental calcium transport (Kovacs et al., 1996).

(IV) Vitamin D Metabolites during pregnancy

25-Hydroxyvitamin D: Plasma 25(OH) D levels in pregnant women have been determined by numerous workers with conflicting results. Many workers (Rosen et al.,1874; Dent & Gupta, 1975, Weisman et al., 1978 a; Weiland et al., 1980) have reported similar plasma 25(OH) D values in pregnant and non-pregnant women. On the other hand, Turton et al.(1977), MacLennan et al. (1980) and Cockburn et al. (1980) have reported lower plasma values of 25(OH) D in pregnant women in the third trimester than in non-pregnant controls. Bedouins in Israel (Biale et al., 1979) and Asian immigrants in the UK (Heckmatt et al., 1980) have shown lowest 25 (OH) D values in pregnancy. Pregnant women in Belgium (Boillon et al., 1977), Switzerland (Paunier et al., 1978) have also reported lower levels of 25(OH) D in pregnancy than their North American counterparts (Steichen et al., 1980). The variations in the reports of 25(OH) D in pregnancy (and even non-pregnant state) may be attributed not only to the latitude of the cities from where these reports have originated but also the variations in the degree of solar exposure and the amount of dietary intake of vitamin D in different populations. Ponson et al., (2010) have reviewed literature on vitamin D status in pregnancy published between 1997 and 2006. They concluded that vitamin D deficiency was common in darkly pigmented mothers particularly those who have migrated to regions with low UV radiations. Vitamin D deficiency was also found to be prevalent in Caucasian women, especially who had not taken vitamin D supplements during pregnancy. Dror and Allen (2010) have also confirmed a high prevalence of maternal vitamin D inadequacy during pregnancy and at delivery in various ethnic populations living at different latitudes.

1, 25-Dihydroxyvitamin D_3: Halloran et al.(1979) have studied vitamin D metabolism during pregnancy in the rat. On day 18th and 20th of pregnancy, 25(OH) D and 24,25 (OH)$_2$ D_3 levels were significantly lower and 1,25 (OH)$_2$ D_3 higher than in non-pregnant control rats. Numerous studies in human pregnancy have also revealed marked rise in plasma concentration of 1,25 (OH)$_2$ D_3 (Weiland et al., 1980; Gertner et al.,1980; Steichen et al., 1980; Boillon et al., 1981). Several longitudinal and cross-sectional studies have shown that, when compared to non-pregnant young women, pregnant women have high serum $1,25(OH)_2D_3$ concentration from early pregnancy; serum $1,25(OH)_2D_3$ concentration rises steadily throughout gestation and reaches levels about double those of non-pregnant women at term (Papapetrou, 2010). The mechanism of increase in plasma levels of 1, 25 (OH)$_2$ D_3 in pregnancy is not exactly clear. The possible mechanisms are through placenta and kidneys. In placenta, 1-α-hydroxylase expression was 80-fold higher in the first and second when compared with the third trimester biopsies. Therefore, if the placenta was the main source of circulating $1,25(OH)_2D_3$, one would expect the level of $1,25(OH)_2D_3$ to be higher during early than late stages of pregnancy. Thus, it seems more probable that the $1,25(OH)_2D_3$ in the maternal circulation originates mainly from the maternal kidneys (Kovacs, 2008; Papapetrou, 2010).

(V) Placental Transfer of Vitamin D and its Metabolites

The importance of placental transfer of vitamin D and its metabolites was suggested almost a century ago by the clinical reports of fetal rickets in offspring of Chinese osteomalacic mothers (Maxwell & Miles, 1925). More recently, neonatal rickets have been reported in vitamin D-deficient Asian immigrants in UK (Ford et al., 1973). In animal studies, vitamin D supplements given to pregnant rats resulted in a delay in the onset of rickets in the pups given rachitic diet at weaning (Korenchevsky & Carr, 1939). Direct evidence of transfer of vitamin D and its metabolites across the placenta in animals was provided by many workers (Haddad et al.,1971; Ross et al., 1979; Barlet et al., 1979; Schediwie et al., 1980). In pregnant sheep, ^{3}H-vitamin D_3 was administered in physiologic doses and maternal and fetal plasma concentrations of ^{3}H-vitamin D and [3]H-25 (OH) D were estimated 19 hours later. ^{3}H-vitamin D and [3]H-25 (OH) D could be detected in the fetal plasma but equilibrium was not observed with maternal plasma levels (Ross et al.,1979). This study demonstrated the permeability of placenta to vitamin D and 25(OH) D. Rapid placental transfer of 1,25 (OH)$_2$ D$_3$ to the fetus has been demonstrated in Rhesus monkey (Schediwie et al., 1980), but not in rat (Noff & Edelstein, 1978). Since vitamin D receptors (VDR) have been detected in the placenta and fetal kidneys, it is possible that fetal 1,25 (OH)$_2$ D$_3$ results from fetal metabolism of 25 (OH) D in the placenta or fetal kidney (Kovacs, 2008).

F.   ROLE OF VITAMIN D IN LACTATION

Lactation presents a calcium challenge to the mother similar to that experienced during pregnancy. In some species, e.g. rat, the stress on the calcium homeostatic mechanisms is far greater in lactation than in pregnancy. In 21 days of lactation, the rat transfers to her litter over 2.5 g of calcium, equal to 60 % of calcium content of her skeleton. The daily loss of calcium in the milk in lactating rat usually exceeds 100 mg which is 100 times more than daily urinary calcium excretion. In human female, calcium loss in milk (350 mg/day) is only marginally greater than the 24-h urinary calcium excretion.

(I)   Intestinal calcium absorption

In the lactating rat, food intake is 3 to 4 –fold greater than in non-lactating rat. The increase in appetite is attributed to suckling induced stimuli as well as metabolic drain of milk production. The structural changes in the jejunum include increase in villus height, crypt depth and total tissue mass (Cripps & Williams, 1975; Burdett & Ruk,1979). The mechanism of intestinal adaptive changes is not clear. Prolactin has been suggested as one of such hormones. Prolactin is a tropic hormone for mammary glands. Similar action in the intestinal mucosa is quite likely (Harding & Cairnie, 1975; Maionoya, 1978).

In vitro preparations, many workers have confirmed increased intestinal absorption of calcium in lactating rats (Kostial et al., 1969 a; Kostial et al., 1969 b; Toverud et al., 1976). In the studies of Fournier & Susbielle (1952) when the diet contained 100 mg calcium per day, calcium absorption in lactating rat was 50% of the dietary intake, as compared to 10 % in controls. When the dietary calcium content was reduced to 27 mg/d in the lactating rats, the intestinal absorption of calcium was almost 100 %.

In view of the well-known action on calcium-binding protein synthesis, increased intestinal absorption of calcium may be attributed to increased plasma levels of 1, 25(OH)$_2$ D$_3$. However, intestinal calcium absorption remains high during lactation even in vitamin D-deficient rats (Toverud et al., 1978). Halloran and DeLuca (1980 b) studied the intestinal calcium absorption by everted gut sac technique. Duodenal sac of lactating rat, which had been deprived of vitamin D for a long time and had undetectable plasma levels of 25(OH) D and 1,25 (OH)$_2$ D$_3$, showed significantly higher calcium absorption than duodenal sac of non-lactating rat. Further, duodenal sac of vitamin D-replete lactating rat showed still higher calcium absorption. From these studies, it was concluded that besides vitamin D, there is a vitamin D-independent component of increased intestinal transport of calcium associated with lactation.

The fractional absorption of calcium (FA-Ca) was measured using a dual non-radioactive Ca isotope technique in 26 control women, 49 women in the last trimester (36 weeks) of pregnancy and 31 of these women in established (20 weeks) lactation. It was concluded that that FA-Ca is significantly elevated in late pregnancy but not in established lactation, when compared with control women (Kent et al., 1991). In contrast to the high 1, 25-dihydroxyvitamin D$_3$ levels of pregnancy, maternal free and bound 1, 25-dihydroxyvitamin D levels fall to normal within days of parturition and remain there throughout lactation. Consequently, the intestinal absorption of calcium is equal to the non-pregnant state and decreased from pregnancy. This change coincides with the fall in 1, 25-dihydroxyvitamin D levels to normal.

While scanning the literature on intestinal calcium absorption in lactation, it would be pertinent to note the species difference in calcium metabolism. In the rat, calcium requirements of the fetus are almost negligible as compared to calcium requirements during lactation. During the last two months of human pregnancy, daily fetal requirement of calcium is greater than calcium secreted in milk (Spray, 1950). This fact may explain why firm evidence of enhanced intestinal calcium absorption is available during pregnancy but not during lactation.

(II)   Urinary Calcium Excretion

In the rat, urinary calcium excretion during lactation appears to be lower than that of pregnant or non-lactating rats. In a study by Fournier & Susbielle (1952), daily urinary calcium excretion decreased from 2 mg during pregnancy to negligible during second and third week of lactation. The decrease in urinary calcium excretion has been attributed to a decrease in plasma calcium level (lowered filtered load), and to elevated plasma PTH level. However, the contribution of reduced urinary calcium excretion to the calcium economy of a lactating rat is negligible.

In non-pregnant, non-lactating women, almost 200 mg calcium is lost daily in the urine. In lactating women, a similar amount is lost in the milk (Toverud & Boass, 1979). Hence a small change in urinary calcium excretion may make an important contribution to calcium balance in a lactating women. The GFR falls during lactation to a level below the pregnant and non-pregnant value, and the renal excretion of calcium is typically reduced to levels as low as 50 mg per 24 h (Kovacs, 2001).

(III)   Bone Metabolism in Lactation

Halloran and DeLuca have investigated bone metabolism during lactation in the rat. On a diet containing adequate amounts of calcium, phosphate and vitamin D, 27% loss of femur calcium was observed during lactation. Whereas vitamin D-replete rats lost 40 mg calcium from the femur during lactation, vitamin D-deficient rat lost 46 mg. Histological examination revealed loss of both cortical and trabecular bone. On the basis of these experiments, it was concluded that although vitamin D is necessary to ensure normal calcium homeostasis during lactation, some other hormonal mechanism promotes bone calcium release.

In human lactation, serial measurements of bone density have shown a fall of 3–10.0% in bone mineral content after 2–6 months of lactation. Trabecular sites (lumbar spine, hip, femur, and distal radius), are affected more than cortical sites (**Kovacs, 1997**). Loss of bone mineral from the maternal skeleton seems to be a normal consequence of lactation and may not be preventable by raising the calcium intake above the recommended dietary allowance. Several recent studies have demonstrated that calcium supplementation does not significantly reduce the amount of bone density lost during lactation (**Polatti et al., 1999)**). Not surprisingly, the lactational decrease in bone mineral density correlates with the amount of calcium lost in the breast milk output (**Laskey et al., 1998**).

The studies of pregnant women suggest that the fetal calcium demand is met in large part by intestinal calcium absorption, which more than doubles from early in pregnancy and possibly the maternal skeleton does contribute calcium to the developing fetus. In comparison, the studies in lactating women suggest that skeletal calcium resorption is a dominant mechanism by which calcium is supplied to the breast milk, while renal calcium conservation is also apparent. These observations indicate that the maternal adaptations to pregnancy and lactation have evolved differently over time, such that dietary calcium absorption dominates in pregnancy, whereas the temporary borrowing of calcium from the skeleton appears to dominate during lactation. Lactation seems to program an obligatory skeletal calcium loss irrespective of maternal calcium intake, but the calcium is completely restored to the skeleton after weaning (Kovacs 2001).

(IV)   Vitamin D Metabolism

A non-pregnant, non-lactating rat has to be deprived of vitamin D for several weeks before hypocalcemia develops. On the other hand, if vitamin D is withheld even after the first week of pregnancy, hypocalcemia may be observed by the middle of lactation period (Halloran et al., 1979; Boass et al., 1981 a). Increased plasma levels of 1, 25 $(OH)_2$ D_3 during lactation were reported for the first time by Boass et al. (1977). Halloran et al. (1979) not only confirmed the elevated circulating levels of 1,25 $(OH)_2$ D_3 in lactating rats but also observed a reciprocal relationship with 24,25 $(OH)_2$ D_3. Hypocalcemia and resulting increased PTH levels demonstrated in lactating rats seem to be responsible for increased renal 1-alpha-hydroxylase activity. Parathyroidectomy in the rat at mid-lactation led to a marked decline in serum calcium and 1, 25$(OH)_2$ D_3 levels. However, factors other than PTH also seem to be involved in increased synthesis of 1, 25 (OH) D_3, since even after parathyroidectomy, serum levels of 1, 25 (OH)2 D_3 in lactating rats were found to be twice that of non-lactating rats (Pike et al., 1979).

In humans, 1, 25 (OH)2 D levels increase 2-3 folds during pregnancy, but within days of delivery fall to normal range and remain so throughout lactation (Wilson et al., 1990).

(V)   Transfer of Vitamin D and its Metabolites in Milk

Vitamin D and its metabolites circulate in blood bound to a specific transfer protein called vitamin D-binding protein (DBP). DBP expresses binding preference for 25 (OH) D as compared to the parent vitamin or 1,25 $(OH)_2$ D_3 (Haddad & Walgate, 1976; Imawari et al.,

1976; Belsey et al., 1974). Level of DBP in human milk is rather low. Compared to average plasma DBP concentration of 525 µg/ml, milk contains only 18 µg/ml at the beginning of lactation which falls to about 3 µg/ml three weeks later (Haddad & Walgate, 1976). Maternal blood levels of various vitamin D metabolites determine the amount of these metabolites in milk. Milk from a mother who is vitamin D-deficient would be devoid of vitamin D and its metabolites. On the other hand, vitamin D content of milk can be increased by administration of a large dose of vitamin D to the mother (Polskin et al., 1945; Hibb and Ponden, 1955). Concentration of 25 (OH) D in milk is stable. Dihydroxylated metabolites constitute an insignificant component of antirachitic properties of milk (Hollis et al., 1981).Since DBP occurring in milk has its origin in the plasma and vitamin D and all of its metabolites bind to the protein, DBP entering milk provides an important route for the transfer of vitamin D and its antirachitic metabolites. Colostrum is extraordinarily rich in plasma proteins (Larson, 1974). Hence, colostrum is particularly rich in antirachitic sterols (Oh & Horst, 1981).

G.   EFFECTS OF VITAMIN D DEFICIENCY DURING PREGNANCY

Liu and Chu (1943) described in detail the effects of vitamin D deficiency in pregnancy. The clinical, biochemical, radiological and histopathological features of osteomalacia in pregnant and lactating women are too well known to warrant repetition (Fourman & Royer, 1968). In babies born to such mothers, neonatal hypocalcemia (Cockburn et al., 1980), and even congenital rickets have been reported (Maxwell et al., 1939; Liu et al., 1940; Snapper, 1956).

The possible role of vitamin D in reproduction has attracted attention during the last few decades. Sunde et al.(1978) observed abnormal embryonic development of chicks, when hens were put on diet deficient in vitamin D. Henry and Norman (1978) reported eggs from vitamin D deficient-hens were practically incapable of hatching. Halloran and DeLuca (1980a) maintained weanling female rats on vitamin D-deficient diet. Such animals showed hypocalcemia and poor growth as compared to vitamin-replete rats. It was found that the likelihood of vitamin D-deficient rats becoming pregnant was only one-half as in vitamin D-replete rats. Moreover, even when the rats became pregnant, only 40% of the vitamin D-deficient females reached full term as compared to 80% incidence in vitamin D-replete rats. Even the mean litter size of vitamin D-deficient rats was 7.8 as compared to vitamin D-replete rats as compared to 11.2 in vitamin D-replete rats. Mean birth weight of each pup was similar in the two groups. Histological examination of fetal tissues did not reveal any abnormality in liver, kidney, brain, or spleen. Miller et al.(1982) reported slight, yet significant, increase in the amount of osteoid in trabecular bone surfaces of the pups born to vitamin D-deficient rats.

Vitamin D deficiency during pregnancy seems to produce adverse effects in the offspring that become more evident during postnatal life. Brommage and Neuman (1981) observed growth retardation in the pups at the age 12-14 days when the mother was deprived of vitamin D during pregnancy. Hypocalcemia, hypophosphatemia and impaired bone calcification was observed by the age of 23 days (Halloran et al., 1979; Halloran & De Luca. 1980 c). Boass et al (1981 a) undertook a systematic study of the effects of short term vitamin D deprivation of the mother from 6th day of pregnancy on the suckling and weaned rat pips. By 15th day, serum (OH) D was undetectable and the body weight was reduced by 26%. Serum calcium and phosphate levels were also reduced. In 19 days old pups, the ratio of bone weight to body weight was not reduced but ash weight as a percentage of body weight was 33% as compared to 36 % in pups from vitamin D-replete mothers. Histological examination of the bone revealed irregularity and widening of epiphyseal cartilage of long bones, a characteristic feature of vitamin D-deficiency rickets.

Brommage and De Luca, (1984 a) tried to determine whether the failure of vitamin D-deficient pups to grow was due to a maternal or neonatal defect. When vitamin D_3 was provided to the pups, there was no improvement in their growth, but administration of vitamin D_3 to vitamin D-deficient mothers produced a three-fold increase in growth rate of the pups. The position was further clarified when vitamin D-deficient mothers were given only two pups to nourish whereas eight pups were nourished by vitamin D-replete mothers. The growth rate was now similar in the two groups. Moreover, using isotope studies, vitamin D-deficient rats were found to produce about 20 % of milk produced by vitamin D-replete rats, On the basis of these experiments, it was concluded that vitamin D-deficient rats produce a reduced quantity of nutritionally adequate milk (Brommage & De Luca , 1984 b).

In human pregnancy, even mild deficiency of vitamin D seems to reduce the fetal growth. In Asian immigrants in the UK, due to low dietary intake of vitamin D and reduced solar exposure, low serum 25 (OH) D levels as well as low serum calcium and phosphate levels have been reported in mothers as well as new born (Heckmatt et al., 1979; Cockburn et al., 1980). Administration of vitamin D to such pregnant mothers resulted in an improvement in serum calcium status of the mother as well as the fetus (Brooke et al., 1980, Maxwell et al.,

1981). In women of Haryana (India), who do not show any evidence of vitamin D deficiency during non-pregnant state (Marya et al., 1981 b), administration of vitamin D supplements during pregnancy produced a dose related increase in birth weight of the babies. Many anthropometric measurements of the new born such as length, head circumference and skinfold thickness also showed improvement (Marya et al.,1981 a; Marya et al., 1988; Puri et al., 1989).

Vitamin D deficiency is common in pregnant women (5-50%) and in breastfed infants (10-56%), despite the widespread use of prenatal vitamins, because these are inadequate to maintain normal vitamin D levels. Adverse health outcomes such as preeclampsia, low birth weight, neonatal hypocalcemia, poor postnatal growth, bone fragility, and increased incidence of autoimmune diseases have been linked to low vitamin D levels during pregnancy and infancy (Mulligan et al 2010).

III. MATERIALS AND METHODS

This study was conducted on 3-4 months old Wistar albino rats weighing 150-175 g obtained from animal breeding center, Haryana Agricultural University, Hisar (India). The rats were put on commercial diet supplied by M/S Lipton India, Calcutta. The rat feed had the following composition:

Crude protein. 21%

Ether extract :   5%

Crude fiber :   4%

Ash :   8%

Calcium: 1%

Phosphorus: 0.6 %

Nitrogen free extract: 55%

Metabolisable energy : 3600 Kcal/Kg

Vitamin D content : 1800 IU/ Kg feed

The rat feed and water were available to the animals ad libitum. The rats were kept away from direct sunlight, in an animal room maintained at 27 ± 1^O C. Soft straw dust provided the bedding and nesting material. Animals were kept in cages of appropriate size.

After maintaining the rats on commercial diet for four weeks, the rats were allowed to mate and fed same diet throughout the experiment. The Harem system of mating (six females and 2 males in a cage) was followed. Every day, vaginal swab of each female was subjected to microscopic examination (Hafez, 1970). Observation of sperms in the vaginal smear was taken as a confirmation of pregnancy in the rat. The pregnant rat was moved to a separate breeding cage and allowed to deliver and nourish the pups till 28th day of age. In each litter, on the 3rd day of lactation, the number of pups was adjusted to eight, so as to equalize the metabolic drain on the mother. The mother was weighed daily during pregnancy and lactation. The pups were weighed within 24-36 hours after birth and subsequently on the 10th (d10), 20th (d20) and 28th day (d28) of age.

To study the various aspects of the effects of vitamin D supplementation in pregnancy and lactation, four series of experiments were performed.

1.   Group A Studies

Vitamin D_3 was administered in three different doses each as a single intra-muscular injection on 10-12th day of pregnancy and the effects on body weight of the mother was recorded during pregnancy on d1 and d21 and subsequently on d1, d10, d20 and d28 of lactation. The pup's weight was recorded at birth, d10, d20, d28. Soft tissue growth and skeletal growth (tibial bone) of the pups were compared with controls on d28. Of 12 pregnant rats given vitamin D_3, only 7 mothers successfully completed the pregnancy-lactation cycle. Others had to be discarded because of abortion in the later part of pregnancy or death of many pups in early neonatal period. Death of pups after 3-4 days of age was not common.

2.   Group B Studies

A large dose of vitamin D administered during pregnancy is known to produce a sustained increase in plasma level of vitamin D and its metabolites during pregnancy and lactation. The passage of vitamin D and its metabolites across the placenta (Ross et al., 1979) and milk (Hibbs & Ponden, 1955) is well known. Therefore, vitamin D administration in pregnancy could have acted during pregnancy as well as during lactation and produced the results observed in the pups at d28 studied in Group A. To differentiate the two aspects, another group of (n=8 each) was administered similar three of vitamin D on the third day of lactation (instead of during pregnancy). The effect on body weight of the mother was recorded on d1, d10, d20 and d28 of lactation. The pup's weight was recorded at birth, d10, d20, d28. Soft tissue growth and tibial bone of the pups was compared with controls on d28. This group of rats was designated "Group B."

3.   Group C Studies

In group A studies, the effect of vitamin D administration in pregnancy on soft tissue growth of the pups was studied only at d28. In order to further explore the effects on soft tissue growth in neonatal period, the effect of vitamin D administration during pregnancy was examined on the soft tissue growth of pups at birth, d10, d20 and d28. This group was designated as "Group C". In this group, 40 rats were administered vitamin D, in a dose that was found to produce optimum growth in the pups at d28 in group A. Six to eight pups were sacrificed each at birth, d10, d20 and d28 and soft tissue growth was studied.

4.   Group D Studies

Administration of vitamin D to the mother during lactation, as done in group B studies, may improve the neonatal growth by improving the lactational perform-ance of the mother or by a direct action on the tissues of the pups. To examine the latter possibility, Vitamin D was administered in a small dose directly to 50% of the pups in each litter of control mothers (10 litters in all), on the 10th day of age. The body weight of the vitamin D supplemented groups was recorded at d20 and 28 compared with that of non-supplemented pups. This part of the study was designated as "Group D" studies.

Investigations in Group A

Vitamin D_3 (cholecalciferol, Duphar-interfran Ltd., Bombay) was administered in three different doses in 100µL of arachis oil (I.P.) as a single intramuscular injection on the 10-12 day of pregnancy as detailed below. The control group of pregnant rats (Group A I) received intramuscular injection of the vehicle on the 10-12 day of pregnancy.

Group A I: 100µL of arachis oil

Group A II: Vitamin D_3 3,000 I.U.

Group A III: Vitamin D_3 7,500 I.U.

Group A IV: Vitamin D_3 15,000 I.U.

(I)   Plasma calcium estimation

On 28th day of age, 3 pups from each litter were sacrificed by decapitation. O.5 ml of blood was withdrawn in a heparinized syringe by intracardiac puncture and used for estimation of plasma calcium level. Similar amount of blood was removed from the mother's tail vein to estimate maternal plasma calcium level.

(II)   Soft tissue studies

The brain, liver and both gastrocnemius muscles were removed from the sacrificed pups, weighed, homogenized and used for the estimation of :

a)   Protein content,

b)   RNA content,

c)   DNA content,

d)   Protein/DNA ratio and

e)   RNA/DNA ratio

(III)   Skeletal Studies

a)   The two tibial bones were isolated from the sacrificed pups and used for the study of dry weight and bone ash.

b)   In 3 additional pups from each sub-group , the right tibia was isolated, decalcified, and used for microscopic examination of the epiphyseal cartilage.

(IV)   Maternal Food Intake

On 14th, 15th, and 16th day of lactation, the daily food intake of the mother was estimated.

Investigations in Group B

In this group of rats were maintained on the commercial diet and allowed to mate. On third day of lactation, vitamin D was administered to the mothers in doses similar to those in group A i.e. Group BI, BII, BIII, BIV received 0, 3,000 IU, 7,500 and 15,000 IU of vitamin D_3. On d28, 3 pups from each litter were sacrificed and investigated for:

(i)   Serum calcium estimation

(ii)   Soft tissue studies

(iii)   Skeletal studies

Maternal food intake was estimated on d14, d15 and d16 of lactation.

Investigations in Group C

In this series of experiments, Group CI, CII, CIII, and CIV received vitamin D_3 in doses of 0, 3,000 IU, 7,50IU and 15000IU of vitamin D_3 respectively on 10-12 day of pregnancy. The pups were sacrificed d1, d10, d20 and d28.

At d1 and d10, all the pups in a litter were sacrificed, and livers and brains of each litter were pooled. At d20 and , only 3 pups were sacrificed for soft tissue studies.

Investigations in Group D

In this series of experiments, rats were kept on commercial diet and allowed to mate and suckle the pups after delivery. On 10 day of age, 4 pups in each litter were administered 500 IU or 1000 IU of vitamin D_3 each. The other 4 pups acted as control groups. Both groups of pups in each litter continued to suckle their mother. Body weight of the two groups of pups was compared at d20 and d28.

Collection and Processing of Soft Tissues

The pups were sacrificed by decapitation. The abdominal cavity was opened and the liver removed. The brain was removed after opening the cranial cavity. In the legs, both gastrocnemius muscles were separated from the other muscles and removed from their insertions. The soft tissues were put in ice-cold normal saline, blotted and weighed immediately. There-after, the tissues were frozen at minus $20^{o}C$ and taken out just before the preparation of homogenate. A ten percent tissue homogenate was prepared in ice-cold phosphate buffered sucrose (0.25 M sucrose in phosphate buffer, 0.05 M, pH 7) using Potter-Elevahjem homogenizer fitted with Teflon pestle. The homogenate was used for the estimation of tissue protein, RNA and DNA.

(I)   Estimation of tissue protein

Protein content of tissue was determined using biuret method (Gornall et al., 1949). An aliquot containing 0.1 ml of tissue homogenate was diluted to 2.5 ml with distilled water. The contents were mixed with 3.5 ml of quantitative biuret reagent. After 30 minutes, intensity of color developed was read at 540 mμ against blank. Bovine serum albumin was used as standard.

(II)   Extraction and Estimation of RNA and DNA

(a)   Extraction of nucleic acids

Nucleic acids extraction and estimations were made according to the method of Schneider (1957). Trichloracetic acid precipitates of the tissue homogenate was washed with five volumes of ice-cold trichloracetic acid (10% w/v). The precipitate was then washed with five volumes of absolute alcohol to remove the lipids. Finally, the precipitate was re-suspended in five volumes of Trichloracetic acid and heated at 90 ° C for 30 minutes. After cooling, the sample was centrifuged. The supernatant was removed and used for the estimation of RNA and DNA.

(b)   Estimation of RNA

Nucleic acids extract (0.5 ml) was diluted to 3.0 ml with distilled water. It was mixed with 3.0 ml of orcinol reagent and heated in a boiling water bath for 20 minutes. Intensity of color developed was read at 700 mμ against blank. Yeast RNA was used as standard.

The orcinol reagent was prepared by dissolving 1.0g orcinol in 100 ml of concentrated hydrochloric acid containing 500 mg of ferric chloride.

(c)   Estimation of DNA

To 2.0 ml of nucleic acid extract, 4 ml diphenylamine reagent was added and the mixture was heated in a boiling water bath for 20 minutes. After cooling, optical density of the color developed was read at 600 mμ. Calf thymus DNA was used as the standard.

Diphenylamine reagent was prepared by dissolving 1.0 g of diphenylamine in 100 ml glacial acetic acid containing 2.75 ml of concentrated sulphuric acid.

(III)   Examination of tibial Bones for Dry weight and Ash weight

Both the tibial bones were removed from each animal, cleaned of extraneous tissue and frozen at minus 20°C. Later on, each bone was thawed, thoroughly cleaned and placed in distilled water for 6 h for removal of any adherent soft tissue. The bone was then made fat-free by extraction first with 100 % ethanol and then with 100 % diethyl ether for 24 h each using a Soxhlet extractor. After drying at 90-100 °C for 48 h, the bone was weighed to obtain dry weight. The bone was then ashed in a muffle furnace at 550-600 °C for 24 h. The ash was weighed.

(IV)　Histological Examination of Decalcified Bone

Soft tissue surrounding the tibia was removed and the bone was fixed in 10 % formal saline. The bone was decalcified in 5% formic acid (formic acid 5ml, formalin 5ml, distilled water 90 ml). After 3 days, the decalcifying solution was checked. The decalcifying solution was changed daily till it became negative for the presence of calcium, indicating that the bone was completely decalcified (Culling, 1974). To test for the presence of calcium, 5 ml of decalcifying fluid was neutralized with N/2 NaOH and then 1 ml of 4% ammonium oxalate was added. Absence of turbidity even after a delay of 5 minutes indicated absence of calcium.

The decalcified bone was neutralized by overnight treatment with 5 % sodium sulphate followed by washing in alcohol for 3-4 hours. Further processing of the tissue i.e. dehydration, clearing and impregnation with paraffin was done in automatic tissue processor (Histokinette). With the help of a rotary microtome, 10 μ thick sections were cut. The sections were stained with Haemotoxylin and Eosin (Culling, 1974).

Estimation of Plasma Calcium

Plasma calcium was concentration was estimated using cresophthalein method (Connerty et al., 1964).

Statistical Method

The data was analyzed using Student's "t" test. P value less than 0.05 was taken as significant.

IV. OBSERVATIONS

GROUP A STUDIES

In this series of experiments, 3 different doses of vitamin D_3 i.e. 3,000 IU (Group AII), 7,500 IU (Group A III) and 15,000 IU (Group A IV) were administered to the rats on the 10th-12th day of pregnancy. The results were compared with non-supplemented control pregnant rats (Group AI).

(I) Maternal Body Weight

During pregnancy, the control rats gained about 70 g weight. By d1 of lactation, their mean body weight was still about 20 g more than at d1 of pregnancy, the rest having been lost due to expulsion of the products of conception (Table I). The maternal body weight observed at d1 of lactation, notwithstanding some fluctuations, was maintained till the end of lactation (d28). Actually, these observations do not reflect any maternal weight-promoting effect of pregnancy and lactation cycle. Age and weight matched females who did not become pregnant gained on the average 27 g weight in 49 days (equivalent to 21 days of pregnancy plus 28 days of lactation).

Table I : Effect of administration of vitamin D_3 in pregnancy on maternal weight during pregnancy and lactation. Values are given as mean $\pm$SE(g).

Pregnancy/lactation day (d)	Control (Group A I)	Vitamin D administration		
		3000 IU (Group A II)	7500 IU (Group A III)	15000 IU (Group A IV)
Pregnancy d 1	177.76±4.93	172.80±5.34	180.80±5.38	180.71±5.13
d 21	244.20±9.10	250.00±10.99	258.40±12.29	255.19±9.93
Lactation d 1	197.57±8.00	192.47±5.65	202.40±8.38	195.98±7.12
d 10	201.59±6.08	203.11±4.34	198.20±11.78	201.10±8.12
d 20	201.87±8.07	200.20±4.31	199.80±7.13	202.72±5.18
d 28	199.41±8.15	193.60±4.91	198.65±7.90	200.17±6.18

$p > 0.05$ in all the supplemented groups at each stage.

n = 6 in each group.

(II)　Weight Gain in Pups

The pups were weighed 24-36 hours after birth, since it was observed that if the pups were handled within 24 h of birth, some, if not all, were killed and consumed by the mother. Mean weight of the pups at d1 was 5.58 g ± 0.09 SE in the control (AI) group. In groups AII (who received 3,000 IU vitamin D) and AIII (who received 7,500 IU vitamin D), the mean weight at d1 was slightly greater than the controls, but the difference was not statistically significant. Subsequently, at d10, d20 and d28, the difference became larger and statistically significant (p. 001). At d28, mean weight of the pups was 24% greater in group in group AII and 31% in group AIII as compared to group AI (Table II). However, the difference in weight of the pups between groups AII and AIII was not statistically significant.

In contrast to groups AII and AIII, mean weight of the pups in group AIV (who received 15,000 IU vitamin D) did not show any improvement over the control group till d28.

Table II : Effect of administration of vitamin D_3 in pregnancy on the weight of the pups during the neonatal period. Each group consisted of 6 litters of 8 pups each. Values are mean ± SE(g).

| Age (days) | Control | Vitamin D administration | | |
| | | 3000 IU | 7500 IU | 15000 IU |
	(Group A I)	(Group A II)	(Group A III)	(Group A IV)
1	5.58±0.09	5.66±0.14	5.72±0.11	5.62±0.11
10	14.58±0.52	17.14±1.02[*]	17.26±0.91[*]	14.89±0.67
20	24.80±1.31	34.28±2.43[**]	34.82±1.33[**]	25.71±1.83
28	37.04±2.20	45.82±2.99[**]	48.52±1.35[**]	36.85±2.10

[*]p < 0.05,　[**]p < 0.001.

(III)　Soft Tissue Studies

The significant increase in body weight of the pups at d28 observed in group AIII was reflected in the soft tissues studied i.e. liver, gastrocnemius muscle and brain.

Liver: In group AIII pups, mean weight of the liver (1.9g± 0.06) was significantly (p. 0.01) greater than that in the control pups (1.63g ± 0.08). The protein content and RNA content were also significantly greater (p. 0.001) than in control group (Table III). Study of other indices of cellular growth revealed that the increase in weight of liver was partly due to increase in cell number (cellular hyperplasia) as shown by a significant increase in DNA content (p. 0.01). It was partly due to increase in cell size (cellular hypertrophy) as shown by significant increase in protein/DNA ratio (p. 0.05). The protein synthetic capacity (RNA/DNA ratio) was also significantly greater in group AIII than in group AI (p. 01).

In group AII pups, liver weight as well as most of the indices of cellular growth were greater than those in the control group, but the difference reached significant level only in protein/DNA ratio and RNA/DNA ratio.

In group AIV, the liver weight, as well as, all other indices of cellular growth was no different from the control group. (Table III).

Table III : Effect of administration of vitamin D_3 during pregnancy on the weight, protein, RNA and DNA content in the liver of the pups at d 28 (mean±SE).

| | Control | Vitamin D administration | | |
| | | 3000 IU | 7500 IU | 15000 IU |
	(Group A I)	(Group A II)	(Group A III)	(Group A IV)
Weight,g	1.63+0.08	1.75+0.07	1.95+0.06 [**]	1.69+0.05
Protein,mg	321.6+15.50	356.80+16.55	416.13+14.06 [***]	337.16+11.93
RNA,mg	32.96+1.75	38.47+2.38	44.66+1.56 [***]	31.91+1.22
DNA,mg	4.34+0.22	4.22+0.15	5.13+0.20 [**]	4.82+0.16
Protein/DNA	73.01+3.00	85.33+4.00 [*]	81.1+ 2.51 [*]	69.87+1.11
RNA/DNA	7.62+0.98	9.15+0.50 [**]	8.51+0.33 [**]	6.69+0.41

[*]p/0.05, [**]p/0.01, [***]p/0.001. n = 18 in each group.

Gastrocnemius Muscle: In the supplemented groups AII and AIII, there was a dose related increase in the weight of the gastrocnemius muscle. In group AIII, the muscle weight was 35% greater than in group AI (p. 0.001). The improvement in total weight was reflected in all the parameters of soft tissue growth i.e. protein content, RNA content, DNA content, RNA/DNA ratio and Protein/ DNA ratio (Table IV) The difference in each parameter was statistically significant. The beneficial effect on growth of gastrocnemius muscle was not seen in group AIV.

Table IV : Effect of administration of vitamin D_3 during pregnancy on the weight, protein, RNA and DNA content in the gastrocnemius muscle of the pups at d 28 (mean+SE)

| | Control | Vitamin D administration | | |
| | | 3000 IU | 7500 IU | 15,000 IU |
	(Group A I)	(Group A II)	(Group A III)	(Group A IV)
Weight,g	0.34+0.01	0.45+0.02 [***]	0.46+0.02 [***]	0.31+0.04
Protein,mg	32.87+1.45	47.40+3.22 [***]	49.82+2.66 [***]	30.08+1.37
RNA,mg	2.87+0.17	4.17+0.20 [***]	4.31+0.27 [***]	2.53+0.11
DNA,mg	0.37+0.01	0.48+0.03 [**]	0.51+0.02 [***]	0.33+0.01
Protein/DNA	86.08+2.55	96.71+2.77 [*]	96.87+2.54 [*]	91.15+3.16
RNA/DNA	7.53+0.26	8.01+0.24 [**]	8.45+0.26 [*]	7.63+0.38

[*] p$<$0.05, [**] p$<$0.01, [***] p$<$0.001. n=18 in each group.

Brain: In groups AII and AIII, the weight of the brain was significantly greater than in group AI (p. 0.01). However, in contrast to 35% greater muscle weight, and 20% greater liver weight in group AIII, the brain weight was only 10% greater than in group AI (Table V). Group AIV also showed significantly greater weight of brain than in group AI (p. 0.01), though this group did not show any increase in weights of liver or gastrocnemius muscle.

Like total weight of brain, protein content, RNA content, and RNA/DNA (protein synthetic capacity) were also significantly better in all the three vitamin D-supplemented groups than in controls.

Table V : Effect of administration of vitamin D_3 during pregnancy on the indices of cellular growth in the brain of the pups on d 28 (mean ± SE).

| | Control | Vitamin D administration | | |
	(Group A I)	3000 IU (Group A II)	7500 IU (Group A III)	15000 IU (Group A IV)
Weight, g	1.22±0.03	1.34±0.02**	1.35±0.02**	1.35±0.02**
Protein,mg	107.75±3.18	121.38±2.15**	120.19±2.79**	116.72±2.66*
RNA,mg	6.71±0.35	8.15±0.20***	8.51±0.32***	8.47±0.27***
DNA,mg	1.39±0.05	1.47±0.04	1.48±0.04	1.37±0.02
Protein/DNA	77.51±3.51	82.61±3.01	81.08±3.17	85.19±3.85
RNA/DNA	4.85±0.24	5.54±0.22*	5.75±0.22**	6.18±0.23***

*$p<0.05$, **$p<0.01$, ***$p<0.001$. n = 18 in each group.

(IV) Skeletal Studies

(a) Dry bone weight and Bone ash weight

Dry bone weight in group AII (75.45 mg ± 2.22) and group AIII (81.56 mg ± 1.87) was significantly greater than in the control group (63.45 mg ± 1.97). Compared to the control group, bone ash weight was also significantly greater in groups AII and AIII. On the other hands, in group AIV, neither dry bone weight, nor bone ash weight was different from controls(Table VI).

Table VI : Effect of administration of vitamin D_3 in pregnancy on the dry weight and ash weight of tibial bones of the pups at d 28 (mean ±SE).

| | Control | Vitamin D administration | | |
	(Group A I)	3000 IU (Group A II)	7500 IU (Group A III)	15000 IU (Group A IV)
Bone weight,mg	63.45 1.97	75.15±2.22**	81.56±1.87***	66.91±2.04
Pup weight,g	37.04±2.20	45.82±2.99*	48.52±1.35***	36.85±2.10
Bone/Pup weight, mg/g	1.71±0.04	1.64± 0.04	1.72±0.04	1.81±0.06
Ash weight,mg	38.12±1.64	42.68±1.57*	48.73±1.78***	40.73±1.50
Ash/bone weight, mg/mg	0.60±0.02	0.56±0.01	0.59±0.01	0.61±0.01

*$p<0.05$, **$p<0.01$, ***$p<0.001$. n=18 in each group.

(b)   Histological Studies

In group AI, haemotoxylin- eosin-stained sections of upper ends of decalcified tibia were examined for any histologic evidence of vitamin D-deficiency rickets. The epiphyseal cartilage showed normal compact columnar arrangement of cartilage cells. Hypertrophic cartilage cells were of normal size. The ossification line was evenly demarcated. The mineralized trabeculae were surrounded by only thin layer of osteoid (Fig. 5). In the supplemented groups AII, AII and AIV, the histologic picture was similar to that of group AI pups.

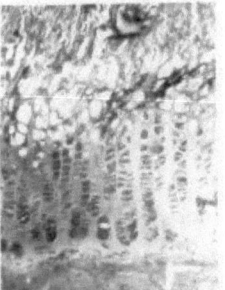

Fig. 5. Histologic section of decalcified proximal tibia from a pup in control group at d28 (H&E stained) (X 200). Normal columnar pattern of epiphyseal cartilage and an even line of ossification can be seen.

(V)   Plasma Calcium Studies

On d28 of lactation, the control group of mothers and pups showed plasma calcium levels of 9.27mg% ± 0.17 and 9.75mg% ± 0.46 respectively. In the supplemented groups, plasma calcium levels both in mothers and pups were practically similar to those in control groups (Table VII).

Table VII : Effect of administration of vitamin D_3 in pregnancy on plasma calcium level at d 28 (mean ± SE mg/dl).

| | Control | Vitamin D administration | | |
		3000 IU	7500 IU	15000 IU
Mothers	9.27±0.17	9.38±0.41[a]	9.41±0.27[a]	9.62±0.41[a]
Pups·	9.75±0.46	9.71±0.47[a]	9.63±0.49[a]	9.55±0.28[a]

[a] p value > 0.05

(VI) Maternal Food Intake

Maternal food intake was estimated on d14-16 of lactation. In these three days, mean daily food intake of the control group was 49.25g ± 1.40. Compared to this, the food intake in the supplemented groups was significantly greater (p. 0.05) in group AII (54. 81g ± 1.69) and AIII (55.16g ± 2.01). Mean food intake in group AIV (47.95 g ± 2.19), however, was not significantly different from than in the control group.

GROUP B STUDIES

In this series of experiments, rats maintained on the commercial diet received vitamin D_3 in three different doses on the third day of lactation.

(I) Maternal Weight

On d1 of lactation, there was no statistically significant difference in the mean body weight of the mothers between the controls (group BI) and groups BII, BIII or BIV who subsequently were injected with vitamin D on d3 of lactation. At d28 of lactation, again, there was no significant difference between the control and the supplemented groups.

Table VIII: Effect of administration of vitamin D_3 in lactation on maternal weight during lactation. Values are given as mean $\pm$SE,(g).

Lactation day	Control (Group B I)	Vitamin D administration		
		3000 IU n = 6 (Group B II)	7500 IU n = 8 (Group B III)	15000 IU n = 7 (Group B IV)
d 1	188.16$\pm$10.52	195.40$\pm$7.65	191.83$\pm$9.10	190$\pm$6.29
d 10	194.33$\pm$7.19	196.80$\pm$8.15	193.65$\pm$10.00	189$\pm$8.57
d 20	195.33$\pm$6.12	205.20$\pm$8.12	193.52$\pm$9.82	197$\pm$8.81
d 28	189.19$\pm$6.92	193.00$\pm$6.13	190.82$\pm$7.21	187.73$\pm$6.15

$p > 0.05$ in all the supplemented groups at each stage.

(II) Weight of pups

On d1 and d10, mean weights of the pups in the supplemented groups were not significantly different from the control group. However, on d20 and d28, mean weights of the pups in group BII and BIII were significantly greater ($p.0.05$) than in control group B1(Table IX). In group BIV, mean weight of the pups was similar to that of controls throughout the neonatal period.

Table IX : Effect of administration of vitamin D_3 in lactation on the weight of the pups. Values are given as mean $\pm$ SE (g).

	Control (Group B I)	Vitamin D administration		
		3000 IU n = 48 (Group B II)	7500 IU n = 64 (Group B III)	15000 IU n = 56 (Group B IV)
d 1	5.92$\pm$0.40	6.02$\pm$0.24	5.94$\pm$0.26	5.95$\pm$0.25
d 10	12.91$\pm$1.00	14.14$\pm$0.72	14.24$\pm$0.48	13.31$\pm$0.89
d 20	22.97$\pm$1.42	27.13$\pm$1.92[*]	27.54$\pm$1.85[*]	22.10$\pm$1.71
d 28	36.89$\pm$2.03	42.97$\pm$2.13[*]	42.80$\pm$2.02[*]	35.13$\pm$2.10

[*]$p/0.05$.

(III) Soft tissue studies

Liver: In groups BII and BIII, at d28, mean weight of the liver was about 16% greater than in the control group BI ($p.0.05$). In the both the supplemented groups, protein, RNA and DNA contents were significantly greater than in control group, indicating cellular hyperplasia (Table X). Protein/DNA ratio and RNA/DNA ratios in groups BII and BIII were similar to those in control group. Group BIV did not show any improvement in liver weight or any parameter of cellular growth.

Table X : Effect of administration of vitamin D_3 in lactation on the weight, protein, RNA, and DNA content in the liver of pup at d 28 (mean ± SE).

| | Control | Vitamin D administration | | |
| | | 3000 IU | 7500 IU | 15000 IU |
	(Group B I)	(Group B II)	(Group B III)	(Group B IV)
Weight,g	1.72±0.08	2.01±0.11[*]	1.98±0.09[*]	1.80±0.12
Protein,mg	341.16±18.22	430.28±17.09[***]	438.00±19.74[***]	359.70±20.13
RNA,mg	31.47±1.70	41.12±1.86[***]	40.93±2.49[***]	34.12± 1.85
DNA,mg	4.45±0.15	5.41±0.22[**]	5.49±0.27[**]	4.89±0.19
Protein/DNA	76.65±2.55	80.31±2.46	79.78±2.06	73.99±2.15
RNA/DNA	7.08±0.26	7.67±0.29	7.45±0.33	6.97±0.47

[*] $p < 0.05$, [**] $p < 0.01$, [***] $p < 0.001$. n = 18 in each group.

Gastrocnemius muscle: Mean weights of the gastrocnemius muscle of the pups in groups BII and BIII were significantly greater than in control group (p.0.05). The protein content, RNA and DNA contents were also significantly greater in these supplemented groups (Table XI). There was no significant difference between these two supplemented groups and the control group as regarding protein/DNA ratio and RNA/DNA ratio. In group IV pups, mean weight of the muscle as well as all indices of cellular growth were essentially similar to the control group.

44

Table XI : Effect of administration of vitamin D₃ in   lactation on the weight, protein, RNA and DNA content in the gastrocnemius muscle of pups at d 28 (mean±SE).

| | Control | Vitamin D administration | | |
| | | 3000 IU | 7500 IU | 15000 IU |
	(Group B I)	(Group B II)	(Group B III)	(Group B IV)
Weight,g	0.40±0.02	0.46±0.01[*]	0.47±0.02[*]	0.40±0.02
Protein,mg	36.91±1.29	41.51±1.06[**]	40.42±1.00[*]	35.73±1.79
RNA, mg	3.34±0.17	3.90±0.19[*]	3.87±0.23[*]	3.60±0.17
DNA, mg	0.36±0.02	0.42±0.02[*]	0.42±0.02[*]	0.36±0.02
Protein/DNA	103.27±3.75	91.70±6.14	101.45±4.10	100.71±4.81
RNA/DNA	9.26±0.36	9.19±0.51	9.04±0.53	9.17±0.72

[*]$p < 0.05$,   [**]$p < 0.01$. n = 18 in each group.

Brain: Mean weight and protein content of brain in groups BII and BIII were significantly greater (p.0.05) than in the control group. All other indices of cellular growth were similar to those in the control group. In Group B IV, brain weight and all other indices of soft tissue growth were similar to those in control group (Table XII).

Table XII : Effect of administration of vitamin D₃ in lactation on the weight, protein, RNA and DNA content in the brain of pups at d 28 (mean ± SE).

| | Control | Vitamin D administration | | |
| | | 3000 IU | 7500 IU | 15000 IU |
	(Group B I)	(Group B II)	(Group B III)	(Group B IV)
Weight, g	1.27±0.03	1.36±0.02[*]	1.38±0.02[*]	1.29±0.01
Protein, mg	108.33±2.28	118.66±2.81[*]	117.14±2.92[*]	108.09±2.17
RNA, mg	6.87±0.24	7.15±0.26	7.39±0.34	6.52±0.28
DNA, mg	1.35±0.03	1.41±0.03	1.42±0.04	1.31±0.03
Protein/DNA	80.34±3.99	83.27±2.85	82.46±3.03	82.44±3.10
RNA/DNA	5.08±0.26	5.07±0.31	5.25±0.27	4.96±0.28

[*]$p < 0.05$ n = 18 in each group.

(IV) Skeletal Studies

In group BII and BIII,(but not group IV) dry bone weight and bone ash weight were significantly greater than in group BI (Control) (Table XIII). Bone weight/pup weight ratio or ash weight/bone weight ratio in any of the supplemented group was not significantly different from control. Histological studies of the epiphyseal cartilage of tibia revealed normal pattern in all the groups.

Table XIII: Effect of administration of vitamin D_3 in lactation on the dry weight and ash weight of the tibial bones of pups at d 28 (mean $\pm$SE).

	Control	Vitamin D administration		
	(Group B I)	3000 IU (Group B II)	7500 IU (Group B III)	15000 IU (Group B IV)
Bone weight, mg	64.85±2.88	77.51±3.07[**]	74.40±3.5[*]	60.18±2.16
Pup weight, g	36.89±2.03	42.97±2.13[*]	42.80±0.02[*]	35.13±2.10
Bone/Pup weight, mg/g	1.76±0.04	1.80±0.04	1.84±0.04	1.71±0.02
Ash weight, mg	37.12±1.84	42.94±1.92[*]	43.10±2.08[*]	35.41±1.42
Ash/bone weight, mg/mg	0.56±0.01	0.55±0.01	0.58±0.01	0.59±0.02

[*] $p < 0.05$, [**] $p < 0.01$. n=18 in each group.

(V) Plasma Calcium

Plasma calcium levels in the mothers and pups at d28 of lactation/age respectively in the supplemented groups (BII, BIII, and BIV) revealed no difference from group BI (Table X IV).

	Control	Vitamin D administration		
		3,000 IU	7,500 IU	15,000 IU
Mothers	9.37±0.27	9.48±0.35[a]	9.41±0.40[a]	9.57±0.28[a]
Pups	9.63±0.38	9.60±0.45[a]	9.87±0.61[a]	9.85±0.52[a]

Table XIV : Effect of administration of vitamin D_3 in lactation on plasma calcium level at d 28 (mean±SE mg/dl).

[a] p Value > 0.05.

Maternal Food Intake

Average daily food intake estimated on o d14-16 of lactation in the control group was 52.07 g ± 1.63. In groups BII, BIII and B IV, mean daily food intake was 55.98 ± 1.17, 56.17g ± 1.81 and 53.87 g ± 1.99, respectively. There was no significant difference in maternal food intake between the control and any of the supplemented groups.

GROUP C STUDIES

In this part of the work, 7500 IU of vitamin D_3 was administered on d10-12 of pregnancy (group CII). Besides total body weight, weight of the liver and brain was estimated in the pups on d 1, d10, and d20. Indices of cellular growth in liver and brain of the pups were also estimated at d1, d10 and d20.

A.   Weight of pups and soft tissues d1-d28

At d1, mean weight of the pups in the supplemented group (CII) was slightly more than in control group (CI), but the difference was not statistically significant (Table XV). At this stage, mean weight of liver of the pups in group CII was not different from group CI (Table XVI). However, mean weight of the brain, even on d1 (Table XVII), in group CII (256 .76 mg) was significantly greater (p. 0.05) than in group CI (220.16 mg). By d10 of age, not only total body weight, but weight of the liver and brain was significantly greater in group CII

47

than in group CI (Tables XV, XVI, and XVII). The difference between the supplemented group and non -supplemented group persisted till d28 (Tables XVIII, XIX, XX and XXI).

Table XV : Effect of administration of 7,500 IU of vitamin D_3 in pregnancy on the weight of the pups during neonatal period. Each group consisted of 6 litters of 8 pups each. Values are mean+SE(g).

Age	Control (Group C I)	Vitamin D administration (Group C II)
d 1	5.64+0.13	5.83+0.10
d 10	15.32+0.65	17.45+0.73 [*]
d 20	23.07+1.61	33.91+1.81 [**]

[*] p<0.05   [**] p<0.001

Table XVI : Effect of administration of 7500 IU of vitamin D_3 in pregnancy on the indices of cellular growth in the liver of pups at d 1 (mean ± SE)n=6 litters each.

	Control (Group C I)	Vitamin D administration (Group C II)
Weight,mg	162.00+17.3	194.25+6.17
Protein,mg	19.51+ 1.95	22.92+0.90
RNA,mg	3.06+ 0.28	3.84+0.41
DNA,mg	0.82+00.09	0.83+0.18
Protein/DNA	23.79+03.66	27.13+3.50
RNA/DNA	3.77+0.27	4.87+0.74

p>0.05 in each.

Table XVII : Effect of administration of 7500 IU Vitamin D_3
in pregnancy on the indices of cellular growth
in the brain of pups at d 1 (mean $\pm$ SE).
n=6 litters in each group

	Control (Group C I)	Vitamin D administration (Group C II)
Weight,mg	220.16+11.51	256.78+10.16[*]
Protein,mg	9.86+ 0.85	12.99+ 0.95[*]
RNA,mg	1.26+ 0.09	1.66+ 0.19
DNA,mg	0.48+ 0.03	0.57+ 0.04
Protein/DNA	20.54+ 1.16	22.47+ 1.00
RNA/DNA	2.61+ 0.21	2.85+ 0.19

[*] $p \underline{/} 0.05$

Table XVIII : Effect of administration of 7500 IU vitamin D_3
in pregnancy on the indices of cellular growth
in the liver of pups d 10 (mean$\pm$SE)n=6 litters
each group.

	Control (Group C I)	Vitamin D administration (Group C II)
Weight,mg	392.16+27.31	486.67+11.16[*]
Protein,mg	50.17+ 2.47	62.22+ 1.61[***]
RNA,mg	6.58+ 0.49	8.17+ 0.45[*]
DNA,mg	1.66+ 0.10	2.27+ 0.20[**]
Protein/DNA	30.24+ 2.82	27.62+ 2.84
RNA/DNA	3.93+ 0.35	3.70+ 0.32

[*] $p \underline{/} 0.05$ [**] $p \underline{/} 0.01$ [***] $p \underline{/} 0.001$.

Table XIX : Effect of administration of 7500 IU vitamin D_3
in pregnancy on the indices of cellular growth
in the brain of pups at d 10 (mean±SE)n=6
litters each group.

	Control (Group C I)	Vitamin D administration (Group C II)
Weight,mg	650.62+17.16	697.75+13.16 [*]
Protein,mg	38.46+ 2.23	41.90+ 2.42 [*]
RNA,mg	3.58+ 0.23	3.65+ 0.25
DNA,mg	1.06+ 0.10	1.18+ 0.16
Protein/DNA	36.32+ 2.29	35.25+ 2.00
RNA/DNA	3.33+ 0.17	3.11+ 0.20

[*] $p < 0.05$.

Pattern of Cellular Growth in Neonatal Period

LIVER: In the control group (CI), the pup weight showed a linear increase throughout the neonatal period. The weight of liver and its protein content also progressive increase till d28. The sharp rise in its weight and protein content during the last week (d20 to d28) was accompanied by a sudden spurt in the cell size (protein/DNA ratio). The increase in cell number (DNA content) was more remarkable during the first 20 days (Fig. 6). Compared to these results, the supplemented group showed basically similar pattern of growth- marked increase in cell number in the first 20 days of postnatal life followed by increased cell size during d20-d28. However, all the indices of cellular growth were greater in group CII than in group CI from d10 onwards (Tables XVI, XVIII and XX).

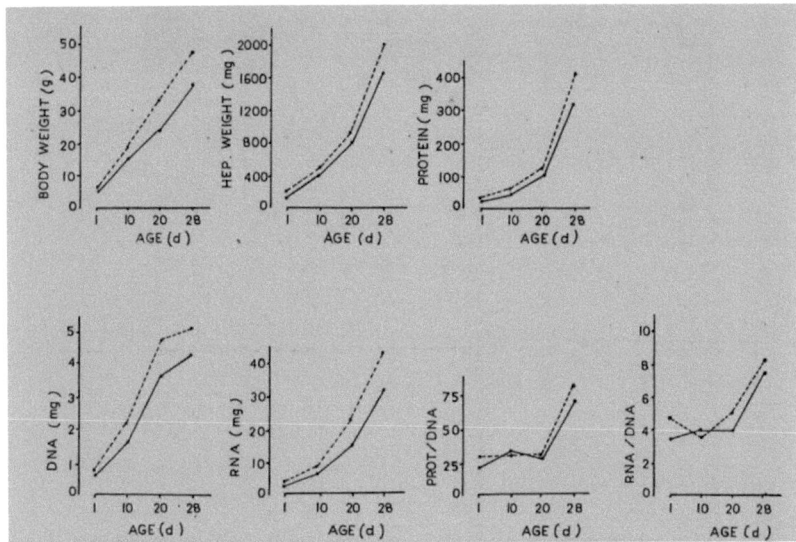

Fig,6.Effect of administration of 7500 IU of vitamin D3 in pregnancy on the pattern of cellular growth in liver of the pups. Control group:_____; Supplemented group:------.

Brain : The pattern of cellular growth in brain was quite different from that seen in the liver. In the control group, the increase in cell number (DNA content) slowed down at d10 and almost ceased at d20. Similarly, increase in cell size (protein/DNA ratio) also slowed down markedly at d20 (Fig.7). Due to these changes, the weight and protein content of the brain increased steeply up to d20 only. In group CII, basic pattern of cellular growth of brain was essentially similar to controls, but the mean weight of the brain was greater than in CI even at d1 and it persisted throughout the neonatal period.

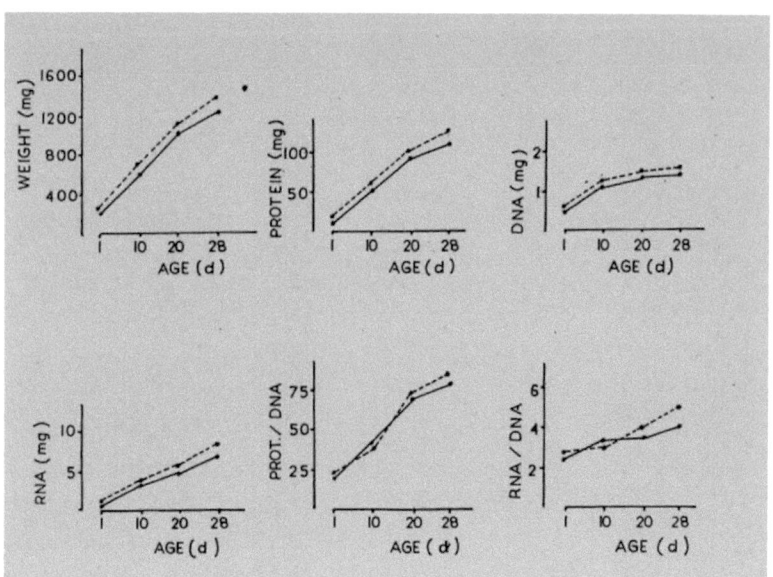

Fig.7.Effect of administration of 7500 IU of vitamin D3 in pregnancy on the pattern of cellular growth in brain of the pups. Control group:_____; Supplemented group:-------

Table XIX : Effect of administration of 7500 IU vitamin D_3 in pregnancy on the indices of cellular growth in the brain of pups at d 10 (mean±SE)n=6 litters each group.

	Control (Group C I)	Vitamin D administration (Group C II)
Weight,mg	650.62±17.16	697.75±13.16 [*]
Protein,mg	38.46± 2.23	41.90± 2.42 [*]
RNA,mg	3.58± 0.23	3.65± 0.25
DNA,mg	1.06± 0.10	1.18± 0.16
Protein/DNA	36.32± 2.29	35.25± 2.00
RNA/DNA	3.33± 0.17	3.11± 0.20

[*] p/0.05.

Table XX : Effect of administration of 7500 IU vitamin D_3 in pregnancy on the indices of cellular growth in the liver of pups at d 20 (mean±SE).

	Control (Group C I)	Vitamin D administration (Group C II)
Weight, mg	760.75±41.07	874.62±18.12[*]
Protein, mg	110.96± 6.80	129.20± 4.61[**]
RNA, mg	15.95± 1.00	23.17± 0.65[***]
DNA, mg	3.80± 0.31	4.75± 0.17[**]
Protein/DNA	28.72± 1.53	27.43± 1.46
RNA/DNA	4.05± 0.30	4.94± 0.32[*]

[*] $p < 0.05$ [**] $p < 0.01$ [***] $p < 0.001$ n=18 in each group.

Table XXI : Effect of administration of 7500 IU vitamin D_3 in pregnancy on the indices of cellular growth in the brain of pups at d 20 (mean±SE)

	Control (Group C I)	Vitamin D administration (Group C II)
Weight, g	1.03±0.03	1.12±0.02[*]
Protein, mg	89.16±3.60	100.70±2.20[**]
RNA, mg	4.91±0.23	5.62±0.20[*]
DNA, mg	1.33±0.06	1.41±0.08
Protein/DNA	66.92±2.10	71.95±1.15
RNA/DNA	3.69±0.35	3.98±0.38

[*] $p < 0.05$ [**] $p < 0.01$ n=18 in each group.

B. Maternal Plasma calcium

As compared to d1, plasma calcium level at d10, 20 and 28, there was slight, but statistically insignificant, decrease in plasma calcium level in both groups CI and CII. There was no significant difference in plasma calcium levels between group CII and CI (Table XXII).

Table XXII : Effect of administration of 7500 IU vitamin D_3 in pregnancy on plasma calcium levels in the mothers and the pups (mean±SE mg/dl)

		Control	Vitamin D administration
Mothers	d 1	9.44±0.28	9.54±0.38[a]
	d 10	9.18±0.35	9.32±0.32[a]
	d 20	9.00±0.26	9.32±0.28[a]
	d 28	9.27±0.17	9.41±0.27[a]
Pups	d 20	9.31±0.41	9.42±0.38[a]
	d 28	9.75±0.46	9.63±0.49[a]

[a] $p > 0.05$.

GROUP D STUDIES

In this part of the study, 500 IU and 1000 IU of vitamin D were administered directly to 50% of the pups of 5 litters each at d10. Comparison of the body of the supplemented groups with the remaining 50% control pups at d20 and d28 did not reveal any significant difference with either dose (Table XXIII).

Table XXIII : Effect of administration of 500 IU and 1000 IU of vitamin D_3 to pups at d 10 on their body weights. Values are mean±SE (g).

Age	Control	Vitamin D_3 500 IU	Control	Vitamin D_3 1000 IU
d 10	13.33±0.80	13.70±0.83[a]	13.54±0.96	14.15±0.62[a]
d 20	24.33±0.54	23.20±0.91[a]	23.98±0.67	22.17±0.85[a]
d 28	36.62±0.96	36.10±1.20[a]	37.54±1.21	36.72±1.41[a]

[a] $P > 0.05$ n=20 in each group.

54

V. DISCUSSION

Many clinical studies have suggested a beneficial effect of vitamin D supplementation in pregnancy on fetal and neonatal growth. Vitamin D supplementation in pregnancy was found to decrease the incidence of low birth weight babies (Brooke et al., 1980; Maxwell et al., 1981). Brooke et al., (1981) observed no significant difference in the mean birth weights of infants born to vitamin D-supplemented mothers and non-supplemented mothers. However, follow up revealed significantly greater weight and height of the babies of the supplemented group at nine months and twelve months of age, even though, neither the mothers nor the babies, received vitamin D supplements postnatal. In a series of publications, Marya and his colleagues reported a dose-dependent increase in fetal birth weight and other anthropometric measurements of the new born (Marya et al., 1981a; Marya et al., 1988; Puri et al., 1989; Kaur et al., 1991). In the present work, the effects of vitamin D supplementation in pregnancy and lactation on the soft tissue growth and skeletal growth of the rat pups have been investigated. Experimental studies have an obvious advantage over community nutritional studies since dietary and environmental conditions can be rigidly controlled only in the former.

In this work, vitamin D supplements were given to pregnant or lactating rats feeding on a commercial diet containing adequate amounts of vitamin D (1800 IU per Kg diet), calcium (1.0 %) and phosphorus (0.6%).

I.   Group A Studies: Effects of vitamin D Supplementation in pregnancy on neonatal growth

In group A studies, groups of rats received vitamin D_3 supplements on 10-12th day of pregnancy as a single intramuscular injection. Group AII received 3,000 IU, group AIII 7500 IU and group AIV 15,000 IU of vitamin D. Group AI (control) received only the vehicle. The dose of 3000 IU vitamin D was roughly equivalent to the amount which was found by the author to produce best results in human pregnancy (Marya et al, 1981a).

(a)   Body weight

Administration of 3000 IU vitamin D in group AII and 7500 IU of vitamin D in group AIII resulted in birth of pups with slightly greater weight than controls, but the difference did not reach significance level. However, by d10, pups in both the supplemented groups were significantly heavier than control. The difference became more prominent by the age d28, when group AII and AIII pups were 24% and 31 % heavier than controls respectively (Table II). These results are comparable with the clinical observations of Brooke et al., (1981) wherein, although the birth weight and length of new born babies of the mothers supplemented with vitamin D during pregnancy was no different from babies of non-supplemented mothers, but the babies of the supplemented mothers were heavier and taller than those of non-supplemented mothers at the age of 9 month and one year.

Administration of a still larger dose i.e. 15,000 IU vitamin D in pregnancy (group AIV) did not produce any beneficial effect on the neonatal growth of the pups (Table II). This observation suggests that over and above the normal dietary intake of vitamin D, administration of only a limited dose of vitamin D during pregnancy produces a beneficial effect on the neonatal growth. Higher doses may not only fail to promote neonatal growth but may even produce actual growth retardation. Administration of 20,000 IU vitamin D per day during pregnancy has been reported to produce severe growth retardation in suckling rat pups (Ornoy et al., 1972).

(b)   Soft Tissue Growth

The well- known target organs for vitamin D include the bone, intestinal mucosa and the kidney. However, reports of nuclear receptor sites in a number of other tissues such as skeletal muscle, heart, brain, skin etc. (Haussler et al., 1968: Stumpf et al., 1979) suggest a widespread action of vitamin D. These reports support the belief of Steenboch and Herting (1955) that vitamin D may have an effect on tissue organic metabolism, of which, improvement in growth is one of the manifestations.

In this work, the effect of vitamin D supplementation during pregnancy on three soft tissues, namely liver, brain and gastrocnemius muscle was investigated. In group AIII, at d28, each tissue weighed greater than in control group. The weight of gastrocnemius muscle, liver and brain was 35% 20% and 10% greater than controls, respectively (Tables III-V). The improvement in tissue weight reached significant level even in group AII in case of brain and skeletal muscle. However, in case of liver, as compared to controls, the improvement reached significant only in group AIII. Administration of still higher dose i.e. 15000 IU vitamin D in pregnant rats failed to produce any beneficial effect on the growth of liver, brain or gastrocnemius muscle (Tables III- V).

From the observations on the effects of vitamin D supplementation during pregnancy on soft tissue growth in the neonatal period summarized above, it is obvious that skeletal muscle showed maximal response, brain the least. Besides environmental factors, tissue growth and development is regulated by a genetic control. In various malnutrition and over-feeding experiments reported earlier, brain showed relatively less variation than skeletal muscle (Rosso, 1977; Winick & Noble, 1967). The relative difference in growth promotion between the three tissues examined in this work could also be due to a difference in the population of receptors for 1, 25 $(OH)_2$ D_3. It has been reported that about 60% of vitamin D or its metabolites injected accumulates in the skeletal muscle and the skeleton (De Luca, 1977).

(c)   Skeletal Growth

In this work, estimation of plasma calcium levels in the pups and their mothers and histologic study of epiphyseal cartilage of the tibiae of the pups has been utilized to establish vitamin D status. Dry bone weight and bone ash weight were used as indices of skeletal growth in the pups.

It is important to know the vitamin D status of the pups in control group AI since, in the presence of hypovitaminosis D in this group, the significance of increase in weight of the pups in group AII and AIII observed in this work would be different. Adequate vitamin D nutrition of the rats was assured by vitamin D content (1800 IU/kg diet) of the commercial diet fed to all the rats including controls. Although, many workers have used greater amounts (Boass et al., 1981a; Toverud et al., 1976), the recommended vitamin D content of rat feed is only 300 IU/Kg diet (Porter, 1963; Hariharan, 1985). The calcium: phosphorus ratio of the rat feed used in this study (1.7:1) was also optimum for minimizing the vitamin D requirement of the rats (Stewart, 1975).

There is 8-10-fold increase in body weight during first 28 days of postnatal life in rat pups. This rapid rate of growth in the neonatal period seems to be responsible for sensitivity of the pups to maternal vitamin D-deficiency. Whereas several weeks of vitamin D deprivation is required to produce rickets in adult rats, even short term vitamin D deprivation in pregnant rats results in all the features of rickets in 25-28 days old pups (Boass et al., 1981 a). Therefore, in the absence of facilities for the estimation of plasma levels of vitamin D and its metabolites, histological study of epiphyseal cartilage becomes a useful tool to assess the vitamin D status of the pups. It may be added that, only a few decades ago, study of epiphyseal cartilage in young rat was a well-recognized method for bioassay of vitamin D (Fourman and Royer, 1968).

In the control group, histological study of epiphyseal cartilage at the upper end of tibia (Fig.5) revealed a normal columnar arrangement of the hypertrophic cell layer and an even line of demarcation. Thus, the characteristic skeletal features of hypovitaminosis D i.e. irregular arrangement of hypertrophic cell layer and an uneven line of ossification or wide osteoid borders (Haltrop et al., 1982) were not seen in the control group of rats. The histological picture of epiphyseal cartilage was similar in pups of all the supplemented groups (AI, AII and AIII). Plasma calcium levels in the mothers and their pups at d28 were similar in all the four groups in group A studies (Table VII). From these observations, it may be concluded that un-supplemented control rats were not vitamin D-deficient.

Another evidence of normal vitamin D status of the pups group AI was the fact that ash weight/ dry bone weight ratio was not less than that in group AIV i.e. pups whose mothers received 15,000 IU vitamin D during pregnancy (Table VI). In hypovitaminosis D, bone weight, ash weight and ash weight/ bone weight ratio tend to decrease. For example, the content of ash as percent of dry bone was reported to decrease from 44.9% in normal controls to 17.7% in vitamin D-deficient *adult* animals (Steenbock, 1924). In another study, in 19 days-old pups of vitamin D-deficient mothers, the ash weight as a percent of dry bone weight was significantly reduced to 33.8% as compared to 36.2% in *pups* of vitamin D-replete mothers (Boass et al., 1981 a).

In groups AII and AIII pups (whose mothers received 3,000 IU and 7, 500 IU vitamin D respectively), the tibial dry weight (75.15 mg ± 2.22 and 81.15mg ± 1.87 respectively) was significantly greater than that in group AI (63.45 mg ± 1.97). The ash weight of tibia in pups in the two vitamin D supplemented groups was also significantly greater than in control group (Table VI). However, estimation of bone ash as a percent of dry bone weight did not reveal any significant difference between control group and groups AII and AIII. All of these results indicate greater osteogenesis in pups whose mothers received 3000 IU or 7500 IU of vitamin D during pregnancy.

Bone weight over total body weight ratio (mg/g) was determined to study the relative effect of vitamin D administration on skeletal and soft tissue growth. In groups AII and AIII, the ratio was not significantly different from control group   (Table VI), indicating that in these groups of rats, skeletal tissue showed improvement in skeletal growth in proportion to the improvement in soft tissue growth.

Improved osteogenesis in pups whose mothers received vitamin D supplements during pregnancy has not been reported earlier. However, there is one report in which administration of 1, 25 $(OH)_2$ D_3 has been shown to increase bone mass in normal adult rat (Larson et al., 1977). Some other evidences also suggest that vitamin D may be involved in bone formation. In cultured rat osteosarcoma cells, 1, 25 $(OH)_2$ D stimulates synthesis of osteocalcin in a dose-dependent manner (Price, 1984). In another study, long term administration of 24, 25 $(OH)_2$ D produced marked and dose-dependent increase in bone volume without producing any hypercalcemia (Nakamura et al., 1988).

Like total body weight, dry bone weight, bone ash weight in group AIV pups   (whose mothers received 15,000 IU vitamin D in pregnancy) were not significantly different from controls (Table VI). Ash weight/dry bone weight and bone weight/total body weight were also not different from controls. Therefore, only a limited dose of vitamin D supplement in pregnancy seems to be helpful in promotion of skeletal and soft tissue growth of the offspring. Administration of massive doses of vitamin D during pregnancy may even impair osteogenesis in the fetus (Ornoy et al., 1968, 1969). Ornoy et al. (1968) estimated ash weight as a percent of wet bone weight, in bones of fetuses whose mothers received 40,000 IU vitamin D per day during pregnancy. The value was 15% as compared to 25 % in controls and 28% in those whose mothers received only 4000 IU vitamin D per day during pregnancy.

Effect of vitamin D supplementation in pregnancy on Lactational Performance

Since the increase in body weight of pups in groups AII and AIII reached significant levels at d10 onwards (Table II), increased lactational performance of the supplemented groups of mothers could be one of the mechanisms of improvement in neonatal growth. Mammary gland is one of the target organs for vitamin D metabolites. In autoradiograms of mammary gland of rats on 6th day of lactation, nuclear concentration of radioactivity was observed in alveolar and ductal cells after injection of tritiated 1,25-$(OH)_2$ D (Narbiatz et al., 1981). The role of vitamin D in lactational performance has also been demonstrated indirectly by severe growth retardation in rat pups following maternal vitamin D deficiency   (Boass et al., 1981 a; Brommage and Neuman, 1981; Halloran and De Luca 1980a). In all these studies, the pups appeared normal at birth but stopped growing well at one week of age onwards. The results have been attributed to a severe reduction in milk secretion (Brommage and De Luca, 1984 a,b). These workers have attributed the decrease in milk production to hypocalcemia since food consumption and milk secretion was increased by self-selection of high calcium diet by vitamin D-deficient lactating rats (Brommage and De Luca, 1884 c).

In this work, milk output could not be measured since accurate measurements of milk secretion require the use of radioactive isotopes of water and potassium (Brommage and De Luca, 1984 b). However, estimation of food intake and total body weight of the mothers during lactation can be used to indirectly assess the lactational performance. Food intake of the mothers was estimated on d14-16 of lactation. In groups AII and AIII, mean daily food intake was significantly greater than in group AI (p. 0.05). In spite of this, all the three groups had similar weight during the four weeks of lactation (Table I). These results indicate greater lactational performance of rats in groups AII and AIII than in group AI.

It may be pointed out that even in control mothers; food intake was markedly greater than in non-pregnant rats of similar body weight. During lactation, food intake increases to a level about 4-folds that of non-pregnant, non-lactating rats. The increased appetite appears to be related to the suckling-induced stimuli as well as metabolic drain of milk production (Toverud and Boass, 1979).

From the results discussed above, it may be concluded that improvement in lactational performance was at least one of the mechanisms by which vitamin D administration in pregnancy increased the neonatal growth of the pups. To explore the possibility of an anabolic action of vitamin D on the fetal and neonatal tissues, groups B, C and D studies were conducted. If vitamin D administration in pregnancy improved the neonatal growth merely by increasing lactational performance, administration of similar doses of vitamin D in early lactation may be expected to be equally effective in improving the neonatal growth. Such a possibility has been explored in group B studies.

(II) Group B Studies: Effects of Maternal Vitamin D Supplementation during Lactation on Neonatal Growth

In group B studies, mothers were administered vitamin D_3 on the third day of lactation. Thus, group BII, BII and BIV received 3,000 IU, 7,500 IU and 15,000 IU vitamin D respectively as a single intramuscular injection. At d1 and d10, mean body weight of the pups was similar in all the groups including the control group BI. At d21 and d28, group BII and group BIII pups were significantly heavier than control pups (Table IX). The increase in body weight was reflected in increased weight of soft tissues (skeletal muscle, liver, brain) as well as in bone (Tables X-XIII). It may be concluded that administration of vitamin D in early lactation also improves neonatal growth possibly by increasing lactational performance. In an earlier study, Djojosoebagio and Turner (1964) observed greater milk yield and greater body weight of suckling pups after administration of vitamin in lactation.

Superficially, results of group A (vitamin D supplementation in pregnancy) and group B (vitamin D supplementation in early lactation) studies seem to be similar and therefore improved neonatal growth of the pups may be attributed to better lactational performance in either case. However, a close scrutiny of the data reveals certain important differences between the two groups. One difference was that administration of similar doses of vitamin D produced greater improvement in group A pups than in group B pups. At d28, group AII and AIII showed 24% and 31% greater body weight than group AI pups. In BII and BIII, the pups showed only 16% improvement over control group BI pups. These results could be explained if it is assumed that vitamin D is more effective in improving lactational performance when administered during pregnancy than in lactation. Although there is no direct evidence in support of this view, the possibility is suggested by the fact that mammary tissue normally undergoes hyperplasia during pregnancy. In addition, receptors for $1,25\text{-}(OH)_2$ D_3 have been reported not only in lactating and non-lactating mammary tissue (Reinhardt and Conard, 1980), but also in anterior pituitary cells involved in secretion of growth hormone (Haussler et al., 1982) and prolactin (Wark and Tashjian, 1982). Moreover, human breast cancer cells in tissue culture have been shown to respond to addition of vitamin D metabolites in the medium by greater DNA synthesis (Freake et al., 1981).

Certain differences in the indices of cellular growth between groups A and B suggest that besides better lactational performance, some additional mechanism is involved in the promotion of neonatal growth in the pups in groups AII and AIII. In groups BII and BIII pups, the soft tissue weight and DNA content of liver, gastrocnemius muscle and brain was significantly more than in Group BI, indicating cellular hyperplasia in the tissues of supplemented groups. In over-feeding experiments, similar cellular hyperplasia has been reported by Winick and Noble (1967). The observations on cellular indices, thus, lend further support to the view that improved lactational performance could explain improved neonatal growth when vitamin D was administered in early lactation (group B). On the other hand, in groups AII and AIII, indices of cellular growth showed besides cellular hyperplasia, cellular

61

hypertrophy as well(increased DNA content, increased RNA content, increased protein/DNA ratio). The increased protein synthesis indicated an additional anabolic action of vitamin D administration. Therefore, it may be concluded that vitamin D administration in pregnancy promoted neonatal growth by increasing not only lactational performance but also by some anabolic action resulting in greater protein synthesis. Such an anabolic action might have occurred during neonatal or intrauterine life of the pups. To clarify this point, 500 IU and 1000 IU of vitamin D was administered intramuscularly to 50% of the pups in each litter on d10, while remaining 50% of the pups acted as controls. All the pups suckled their mother who did not receive any vitamin D supplement during pregnancy or lactation (group D studies). At d28, no significant difference could be detected between the weight of vitamin D-supplemented and non-supplemented pups (Table XXIII). These results suggest that anabolic effect of vitamin D occurs only when additional quantity of the vitamin reaches the pups during intrauterine life, but not during postnatal life.

The possibility of a fundamental role of vitamin D in intrauterine growth and development is suggested by the reports of vitamin D receptors in many fetal tissues such as placenta, bone, skin, kidney, yolk sac etc. (Haussler, 1986). The placenta can not only transport vitamin D and its metabolites to the fetus (Haddad et al., 1971;Ross et al, 1979) but also can convert 25(OH)D to 1,25 (OH)$_2$ D (Tanaka et al., 1978). However, it may be argued that if anabolic action of vitamin D on the tissues begins to operate during intrauterine life, why greater birth weight was not observed in group AII and AIII pups? In this regard, it would be pertinent to point out that administration of vitamin D supplements in pregnant women have resulted in greater birth weight (Marya et al.,1981 a, 1988). In rat, the beneficial effect was apparent on d10 only. Probably, the difference lies in the extent to which fetus completes its growth at birth. Mean birth weight of pups at birth is about 2% of its adult weight, whereas a human newborn weighs about 5% of the adult weight. More important differences have been reported between these two species regarding the pattern of cellular growth during intrauterine life and early neonatal period. According to Winick et al. (1972), cellular growth is characterized by three consecutive and somewhat overlapping phases. During the first phase, an organ grows exclusively by increasing its cell number. This phase is reflected by linear increase in DNA content of the organ without change in protein/DNA ratio. In the second phase, rate of cell division falls and cell size begins to increase. Finally, in the third phase cell division ceases and organ growth becomes a function of increase in cell size (increased protein/DNA ratio). In human fetus, rapid increase in DNA content of liver, gastrocnemius muscle, kidney and heart occurs during the first 25 weeks of gestation, after which the proliferative phase slows down. In these organs, protein/DNA ratio begins to increase rapidly during the last 10 weeks of intrauterine life (Widdowson et al., 1972). In the rat, on the other hand, the proliferative phase extends not only throughout intrauterine life but also to the first month of postnatal life (Winick and Nobel, 1965). The only exception is the brain, where the proliferative phase is mostly completed by 20th postnatal day, and liver, where it extends into 48th postnatal day (Winick et al. (1972). Therefore, in the rat, the pattern of cellular growth in the perinatal period is such that alterations in growth process set into motion during intrauterine life are likely to manifest postnatal. The study of the effects of vitamin D administration in pregnancy on the phases of cellular growth studied during the first month of life (group C studies) provide further evidence of intrauterine anabolic action of vitamin D.

(III) Group C Studies: Effects of vitamin D Supplementation in pregnancy on the indices of Cellular Growth at Birth and in first month of Postnatal life

In this series of experiments, 7,500 IU vitamin D was administered to rats on 10-12 day of pregnancy (group CII) and pups were sacrificed at d1, d10, d20 and d28 and indices of cellular growth were studied in the liver and brain.

In group CII, on d1, neither total body weight nor liver weight was significantly different from control group (CI). Only brain weight was significantly greater in group CII. On d10, besides greater total body weight, weight of liver and brain was significantly greater in group CII than in group CI (Tables XV-XX). Comparison of the weight of liver and brain at d1 and d28 in the control group reveals an interesting feature of their growth in perinatal period. At d1, mean weight of the liver (162 mg) was 10 % of the weight at d28 (1.63 g). On the other hand, mean weight of the brain at d1 (220mg) was 18% of the weight at d28. In other words, as compared to liver, a larger percentage of total growth of brain occurs in intra-uterine life. Therefore, anabolic effect of vitamin D, if any, is more likely to manifest at birth in brain rather than in liver.

In the control pups, the pattern of cellular growth in the liver during the first 28 days postnatal was characterized by a marked increase in DNA content till d20 followed by a marked increase in protein/DNA ratio during d20-28 (Fig. 6). Thus, the control group pups

63

showed the usual pattern of cellular proliferation and subsequent cellular hypertrophy. Comparison of this pattern in group CII pups (Fig. 6) showed that vitamin D administration during pregnancy did not alter the basic pattern of cellular growth in the liver. It accentuated the phase of cellular hyperplasia during the first 20 days and extended it till d28. In addition, it produced a larger increase in protein synthetic capacity so that at d28, protein/DNA ratio was significantly greater in the supplemented group.

In the brain (Fig.7), the pattern of cellular growth in group CII was essentially similar to that of group CI, except that all the indices were slightly greater in the former. Some of the indices were significantly greater in group CII even at birth (weight and protein content) while other (RNA content and RNA/DNA ratio) were found to be greater at d28 only.

From the observations on the pattern of cellular growth during the neonatal period discussed above, it may be concluded that additional amount of vitamin D made available during pregnancy modified the tissue growth so as to promote both cellular hyperplasia and hypertrophy but the results manifested chiefly during neonatal period when these processes reached their peak in the rat. However, it remains to be explained how vitamin D could alter the rate of cellular proliferation and protein synthesis.

The role of Ca^{++} in the regulation of cellular proliferation and differentiation has been demonstrated by many workers. Whitfield et al.(1980) observed blockade of DNA synthesis in regenerating liver cells after parathyroidectomy, which could be reversed by calcium supplementation. In mouse epidermal cells, the rate of cellular proliferation and differentiation could be modified by altering Ca^{++} concentration of the medium (Henning et al., 1980). On the basis of such reports, it has been proposed that vitamin D, by regulating intracellular calcium ion concentration may be involved in regulation of cellular proliferation and differentiation (Haussler et al.,1985). In view of the key role of calcium in many exocrine secretions including secretion of milk (Smith et al., 1982; Bhattacharjee et al., 1987), the improved lactational performance in vitamin D supplemented mothers can also explained. Moreover, many studies have demonstrated maximum cellular proliferation at a particular Ca^{++} concentration. Both lower and higher Ca^{++} concentrations decreased the rate of cellular proliferation (Eckl et al., 1987;Boynton et al., 1977). Therefore, it is not difficult to understand why in this work, administration of 3000 IU and 7500 IU of vitamin D improved the neonatal growth of the pups, but 15,000 IU did not.

To conclude, results of this study have demonstrated that in rats on normal intake of vitamin D, calcium and phosphorus, administration of a limited supplement of vitamin D during pregnancy produced a beneficial effect on fetal and neonatal growth. The improvement in growth involved both the skeleton and soft tissues. The accelerated neonatal growth was partly due to an improvement in lactational performance of the vitamin D-supplemented mothers. In addition, certain evidences suggest an anabolic action of vitamin D on the offspring which begins during pregnancy and extends into neonatal period.

VI. SUMMARY

Reports of receptors for $1, 25 (OH)_2 D_3$ in most of the tissues of the body suggest that vitamin D may have a more fundamental and generalized role rather than merely in calcium homeostasis. Many clinical studies, including a few by the author, have indicated a beneficial effect of vitamin D supplementation during pregnancy on the fetal and neonatal growth. The present experimental study was conducted to elucidate the effects of vitamin D supplementation during pregnancy on the skeletal and soft tissue growth in the rat pups.

Throughout pregnancy and lactation, female rats were fed a commercial diet adequate in vitamin D, calcium and phosphorus. Moderate supplements of vitamin D_3 were administered or their pups in four series of experiments. Plasma calcium levels and histological study of the epiphyseal cartilage indicated that control groups of rats were not vitamin D-deficient.

Group A studies: in this experiment, three different doses of vitamin D_3 were administered as a single intramuscular injection on 10-12th day of pregnancy:

Group AI   Control

Group AII   3,000 IU

Group AIII   7,500 IU

Group AIV   15,000 IU

The pups were sacrificed at d28 of age. Estimations of dry bone weight and bone ash weight were used as indices of skeletal growth. Soft tissue growth was studied in the liver , brain and gastrocnemius muscle. In these soft tissues, the pattern of cellular growth was investigated by estimation of tissue weight, protein content, RNA content, DNA content, protein/DNA ratio and RNA/DNA ratio. Maternal food intake was estimated on d14-16 of lactation.

Group B studies: In this experiment, mothers were supplemented with three different doses of vitamin D_3 as a single intramuscular injection on the third day of lactation as follows:

Group BI   Control

Group BII   3,000 IU

Group BIII   7,500 IU

Group BIV   15,000 IU

At d28, the pups were sacrificed and skeletal and soft tissue growth was studied as in group A experiment.

Group C studies: In this experiment, mothers in the experimental group (CII) were 7500 IU of vitamin D_3 as a single intramuscular injection on 10-12th day of pregnancy and pups were sacrificed at d1, d10, d20 and d28. The pattern of cellular growth was studied in the liver and brain.

Group D studies: In this experiment, 500 and 1000 IU of vitamin D were administered directly to the pups at d10 of age. Their body weight at d 20 and d28 was compared with non-supplemented groups of pups.

Observations

The pups in group AII and AIII (whose mothers received vitamin D 3000 and 7500 IU respectively) on d10, d20 and d28 weighed significantly more than the controls.

At d28, mean weight of the liver, brain and gastrocnemius muscle was significantly greater than controls. Indices of cellular growth in each of the soft tissue indicated increases hyperplasia as well as hypertrophy at d28, especially in group AIII.

At d28, dry bone weight and bone ash weight of tibiae in groups AII and AIII were significantly greater than in controls, indicating improvement in skeletal growth in the supplemented groups. However, bone/body weight ratio and ash weight/dry bone ratio in the pups in supplemented was no different from controls.

Mean daily food intake in mothers in group AII and AIII, measured on d14-16 of lactation was significantly greater than controls. In spite of this, mean body weight of mothers in group AII and AIII was not significantly different from group AI. This observation indicated better lactational performance in the supplemented groups. From the results described so far, it was concluded that vitamin D supplementation in pregnancy improved neonatal growth of the pups, at least in part, by increasing lactational performance of the mother.

Supplementation of vitamin D_3 in early lactation (group B studies) also produced a significant increase in weight of the pups in BII and BIII at d20 and d28. However, as compared to as compared to control (BI) pups, the increase in the weight of pups in group BII and BIII was only 16% as compared to 24% and 31% increase in body weight of the pups observed in group AII and AIII. Weight of dry bone and bone ash as well as weights of liver, brain and gastrocnemius muscle in pups of groups BII and BIII were more than in group BI, but the increase in all of these weights were not as much as observed in group I studies.

From the results described so far, it is apparent that neonatal growth of the pups could be increased by administration of vitamin D supplement not only in pregnancy (group A studies), but also in early lactation (group B studies). However, the beneficial effect was more pronounced in the former groups of pups. Besides this difference, there were other qualitative differences between the two studies. In group AII and AIII, vitamin D increased soft tissue growth by promoting cellular hyperplasia and cellular hypertrophy. An increase in cellular protein synthetic capacity was also observed. In BII and BIII pups, the increase in soft tissue growth could be attributed mainly to cellular hyperplasia only. This observation was further supported by observations in group C studies.

Study of the pattern of cellular growth in the liver and brain at d1, d10, d20 in the control pups (group CI) revealed the usual pattern of cellular growth i.e. an initial phase of cellular proliferation followed by a phase of cellular hypertrophy. The proliferative phase (increased DNA content) lasted up to d10 in brain, but continued beyond d20. In the supplemented group, cellular growth in liver and brain followed a similar, but accentuated pattern.

Administration of vitamin D directly to the pups (group D studies) at d10 of age did not produce any improvement in neonatal growth.

To conclude, results of this study have demonstrated that in the rat on normal intake of vitamin D, calcium and phosphorus, administration of a limited supplement of vitamin D during pregnancy produced a beneficial effect on the fetal and neonatal growth. The increase in growth involved both skeletal and soft tissues. The accelerated growth was partly due to an improvement in lactational performance of the mother. In addition, certain evidences suggest an anabolic action of vitamin D on the offspring which begins during gestation and extends into neonatal period.

.

VII.BIBLIOGRAPHY

Adams JS, Clemens TL, Parrish JA, Holick MF 1982 Vitamin D synthesis and metabolism after ultraviolet irradiation of normal and vitamin D –deficient subjects. N Engl J Med 306:722.

Amento EP, Bhalla AK, Kurnick JT, Karadin RL et al. 1984 1,25 –dihydroxyvitamin D_3 induces maturation of human monocyte cell line U 937, and in association with a factor from humn T lymphocytes, augments production of monokine, mononuclear cell factor. J Clin Invest 73:731

Anderson PH, May BK, Morris HA. 1998 Vitamin D metabolism: New concepts and clinical applications. Clin Biochem Rev 24:13-26.

Armato U, Andreis PG, Whitfield JF 1983 The calcium dependence of the stimulation of neonatal rat hepatocyte DNA synthesis and division byepidermal growth factor, glucagon and insulin. Chem Biol Interact 45:203

Askew FA, Bourdillon RB, Bruce HM, Jenkins RGC, Webster TA 1930 The distillation of vitamin D. Proc Roy Soc-B 107:76

Baksi SN, Kenny AD 1977 Vitamin D metabolism in immature Japanese quail: effects of ovarian hormones. Endocrinology 101: 1216.

Baksi SN, Kenny AD, Galli-Gallardo SM, Pang PKT 1978 Vitamin D metabolism in bullfrogs and Japanese quails: effects of estradiol and prolactin. Gen Comp Endocrinol 35:258.

Barlet JP, Davicco MJ, Lefaivre J, Carriolo BJ 1979 Fetal blood calcium response to maternal hypercalcemia induced in the cow by calcium infusion or by Solanum glaucophyllum. Horm Metab Res 11: 57.

Barlett JP, Davico MJ, Lefaivre J, Garel JM 1978 Endocrine regulation of plasma phosphate in sheep foetus with catheters implanted in utero. In: Homeostasis of Phosphate and other Minerals. Ed. Massry GC et al. New York Plenum Press, pp243.

Belsey R, Clark MB, Bernat M, et al.1974 The physiologic significance of plasma transport of vitamin D and metabolites. Am J Med 57:50.

Bhattacharjee M, Weintroub S, Vonderhaar BK 1987 Milk protein synthesis by mammary glands of vitamin D-deficient mice. Endocrinology 121:865.

Biale Y, Levi M, Shainkin- Kestenbaum P, Berlyne GM 1979 25-dihydroxycholecalciferol levels in Bedouin women in labour and in cord blod of their infants. Am J Clin Nutr 32:2380.

Bikle DD, Munson S 1985 1,25-dihydroxyvitamin D increases calmodulin binding to specific proteins in the chick duodenal brush border membrane J Clin Invest 76:2316.

Bickle DD, Nemanic EA, Gee A, Elias P 1986 1,25-dihydroxyvitamin D_3 production by human keratinocytes : kinetics and regulation. J Clin Invest 78:557-566

Boass A, Ramp WK, Toverud SU 1881 a Hypocalcemic, hypophosphatemic rickets in rat pups suckling vitamin D deprived mothers. Endocrinology 109:505

Boass A, Toverud, WK, McCain JW, Haussler MR 1981   Elevated serum levels of 1,25-dihydroxycholecalciferol in lactating rats. Nature 267:630.

Boass A, Toverud WK, Pike JW, Haussler MR 1981 b Calcium metabolism during lactation: enhanced intestinal calcium absorption in vitamin D-deprived, hypocalcemic rats. Endocrinology 109:900.

Bouillon R, Moore P 1973 Pathophysiological data obtained with radioimmunoassay for human parathyroid hormone. Ann Endocrinol 34:657.

Bouillon R, Van Baelen H 1981 Transport of vitamin D: significance of free and total concentrations of the vitamin D metabolites Calcif Tissue Int 33:451.

Bouillon R, Van Baelen H, De Moore P 1977 The measurement of the vitamin d-binding protein in human serum. J Clin Endocrinol Metab 45:225.

Bouillon R, Van Baelen H, Rombaut H, De Moore P 1978 The isolation and characterization of the vitamin D-protein from rat serum J Biol Chem 253: 4426.

Boyle IT, Gray RW, De Luca HF 1971 Regulation by calcium of in vivo synthesis of 1,25-dihydroxycholecalciferol and 24, 25-dihydroxychole-calciferol. Proc Natl Acad SCi USA 68:2131.

Boyle IT, Miravet L, Gray RW, Holick MF, De Luca HF 1972 The response of intestinal calcium transport to 25-hydroxy and 1,25-dihydroxyvitamin D in nephrectomised rats. Endocrinology 90:605.

Boynton AL, Whitfield JF, Issac RJ, Tremblay R 1977 The different extracellular calcium requirement for proliferation of non-neoplastic and neoplastic mouse cells. Cancer Res 37:2657.

Braithwaite GD, Glascock RF, Riaziddin S 1970 Calcium metabolism in pregnant ewes. Br J Nutr 24:661.

Breslau NA, Mc Guire JL, Zerents JE et al 1984 Hypercalcemia associated with increased serum calcitriol levels in three patients with lymphoma. Ann Intern Med 100.1.

Brommage R, De Luca HF 1984 a A maternal defect is responsible for growth failure in vitamin D-deficient rat pups. Am J Physiol 246: E 216.

Brommage R, De Luca HF 1984 b Vitamin D-deficient rats produce reduced quaniies of a nutritionally adequate milk. Am J Physiol 256 : E 221.

Brommage R, De Luca HF 1984 c Self-selection of a high calcium diet by vitamin D-deficient lactating rats increases food consumption and milk production. J Nutr 114: 1377.

Brommage R, Neuman WF 1981 Growth failure in vitamin d-deficient rat pups. Calcif Tissue Int 33: 277.

Brooke OG, Brown IR, Bone CD, et al., 1980 Vitamin D supplements in pregnant Asian women: effects on calcium status and fetal growth. Br Med J 280: 751.

Brooke OG, Butters F, Wood G 1981 Intrauterine vitamin D nutrition and postnatal growth in Asian infants. Br Med J 283: 1024.

Bruns MEH, Fausto A, Alvioli LV 1978 Placental calcium binding protein in rats. J Biol Chem 253: 3186.

Brunvand L, Quigstad E, Urdal P, Huah E. Vitamin D deficiency and fetal growth. Early Hum Dev 1996; 45: 27-33.

Burdett K, Ruk C 1979 Adaptation of small intestine during pregnancy and lactation. Biochem J 184: 245.

Cantorna MT, Hayes CE, DeLuca HF 1996 1,25-Dihydroxyvitamin D3 reversibly blocks the progression of relapsing encephalomyelitis. Proc Natl Sci USA 93: 7861.

Carttar MS, McLean FC, Urist MR 1950 The effect of calcium and phosphorus content of diet upon the formation of bone. Am J Path 26: 307.

Cashard WG, Creditor MA, Canterbury JM, Reiss E 1972 Physiological hyperparathyroidism in pregnancy. J Clin Endocrinol 34: 767.

Chan GM, Buchino JJ, Mehlhorn, D et al 1979 Effect of vitamin D on pregnant rabbits and their offspring. Ped Res 13: 121.

Cherotow BS, Sivitz WI, Baranetsky NG, Clark A, DeLuca HF. 1983 Cellular mechanisms of insulin release. The effect of vitamin D deficiency and repletion. Endocrinology. 1983; 113: 1511.

Cherotow BS, Sivitz WI, Barenetsky MG, DeLuca HF 1986 Islet insulin release and net calcium retention in vitro in vitamin D-deficient rats. Diabetes 1986; 35:771

Clemens TL, Adams JS, Horiuchi N et al 1983 Comparison of 1,25-dihydroxyvitamin D3 receptor binding in keratinocytes and fibroblasts from skin of normal subjects and a subject with vitamin D-dependent rickets. J Clin Endocrinol 56: 824.

Clemens, TL, Zhou XY, Pike JW, Haussler MR, Sloviter RS 1985 1,25-dihydroxyvitamin D recptor and vitamin D-dependent calcium binding protein in rat brain. In: Vitamin D: Chemical, Biochemical and Clinical Update. Ed Norman et al. Walter de Gruyter, pp 95.

Cockburn F, Belton NR, Purvis RJ et al.1980 Maternal vitamin D intake and mineral metabolism in mothers and their new born infants. Br Med J 281:11.

Connerty H, Briggs AR 1964 Determination of serum calcium by means of orthocresolphthalein complexone. Am J Clin Path 45: 290.

Cripps AW, Williams VJ 1975 The effect of pregnancy and lactation on food intake, gastrointestinal anatomy and absorptive capacity of the small intestine in albino rats. Br J Nutr 33:17.

Culling CFA 1974 Handbook of histological and histochemical techniques. London, Butterworth, pp 63.

Davies M, Mawer EB, Hayes ME, Lumb GA 1985 Abnormal vitamin D metabolism in Hodgkins's lymphoma. Lancet 1:1186.

Dawood A, Wagner CL 2007 Mother child vitamin D deficiency: an international perspective. Arch Dis Child. 2007;92:737

Delorme M, Marche P, Garel JM, 1979 Vitamin D-dependent calcium binding protein. Changes during gestation, prenatal and postnatal development in rats. J Dev Physiol 1:131.

DeLuca HF 1971 Active compounds In: The vitamins: chemistry, Physics, Pathology Methods. Ed. Sabrell WH Jr and Harris RS. New York, Academic, 1971; p : 223-232.

De Luca HF 1977 Vitamin D metabolism. Clin Endocr Supple &:1.

De Luca HF, 1984 The metabolism, physiology and function of vitamin D, In: Vitamin D: Basic and clinical aspects Ed Kumar R, Boston, Martinus Nijhoff. Pp 1.

DeLuca HF, Schnoes HK. Metabolism in mechanism of action of vitamin D_3 1976 Annu Rev Biochem. 45: 631.

Dent CE Gupta MM 1975 Plasma 25-hydroxy vitamin D levels during pregnancy in Caucasians and vegetarian and non-vegetarian Asians. Lancet ii:1057.

Denzie D, Boyne AW, Dalgarno AC, et al.1955 Studies of skeleton of the sheep: The effect of different levels of dietary calcium during pregnancy and lactation on individual bones. J Agric Sci 46:425.

De-Regil LM, Palacious C, Ansary A, Kuller R, Pablo P. Vitamin D supplementation for women during pregnancy. Cochrane Database of Systematic Review. 2012 Issue 2 Art. No. CD 008873.

Djojosoebagio S, Turner CV 1964 Effect of parathyroid extract, dihydrotachysterol (Hytakerol) and calciferol on milk secretion in rats. Endocrinology 74:554.

Dokos S, Donaldson CA, Marion SL, Pike JW, Haussler MR 1983 The ovary: a target organ for 1, 25-dihydroxyvitamin D_3. Endocrinology 112:200.

Dostal LA, Toverud SU 1983 Effect of high doses of vitamin D3 and 1,25-dihydroxyvitamin D3 in lactating rats on milk composition and calcium homeostasis of suckling pups. Endocrinology 112: 1631.

Dusso AS, Brown JA, Slatopolsky, E 2005 Vitamin D. AJP Renal Physiology 298:E8.

Eckl PM, Whitcomb WR, Michaloponlog G, Jirtle RL 1987 Effect of EGF and calcium on adult parenchymal hepatocyte proliferation. J Cell Physiol 132: 363.

Fleischman AR, Rosen JF, Cole J, Smith CM, De Luca HF 1980 Maternal and fetal serum 1,25-dihydroxyvitamin D levels at term. J Pediatr 97:640.

Ford JA, Davidson DC, McIntosh WB, Fyfe WM, Duningham MG 1973 Neonatal rickets in Asian immigrant population. Br Med J iii:211.

Fourman P, Royer P 1968 Calcium metabolism and bone, Oxford, Blackwell, pp:112.

Fournier P Susbielle H 1952. Cited by Toverud et al.(1976).

Fraser DR 1980 The physiological economy of vitamin D. In : Pediatric diseases related to calcium. Ed De Luca HF New York, Elsevier. pp59.

Fraser DR, Kidicek E 1970 Unique biosynthesis by kidney of a biologically active vitamin D metabolite. Nature 228:764.

Freake HC, Marcocci C, Iwasaki J, MacIntyre I 1981 1,25 dihydroxyvitamin D3 specifically binds to human breast cancer cell line (T47D) and stimulates growth. Biochem Biophys Res Commun 101:1131.

Func C 1912 The etiology of deficiency diseases. J State Med ;341-348.

Garabedian M, Holick MF, DE Luca HF 1972 Control of 25-hydroxycholecalciferol metabolism by parathyroid glands. Proc Natl Acad Sci USA 69:673.

Garabedian M, Tanaka Y, Holick MF, De Luca HF 1974 Response of intestinal calcium transport and bone calcium mobilization to 1,25-dihydroxyvitamin D3 in thyroparathyroidectomized rats. Endocrinology 94:1022.

Gertner JM, Glassman MS, Coustan DR, Goodman DBP 1980 Fetomaternal vitamin D relationship at term. J Pediatr 97:637.

Gillette ME, Insogna KL, Lewis AM, Baran DT 1982 Influence of pregnancy on immunoreactive parathyroid hormone levels. Calcif Tissue Int 34:9.

Gornall AG, Bardawill CJ, David NM 1949 Determination of serum proteins by means of biuret reaction. J Biol Chem 177:751.

Gray TK 1981 A modified radioimmunoassay for 1,25-dihydroxychole calciferol. Clin Chem 27:458.

Gray R, Boyle I, DeLuca HF 1971 Vitamin D metabolism: The role of kidney tissue. Science 172:1232.

Gray TK, Cohen MS, 1985 Vitamin D, phagocyte differentiation and immune function. Surv Immunol Res 4:200.

Greer FR, Searey JE, Levin RS, et al. 1981 Bone mineral content and serum 25-hydroxyvitamin D concentration in breast-fed infants without supplemental vitamin D. J Pediatr 100:919.

Haddad JG, Birje SJ 1975 Widespread binding of 25 hydroxycholecalciferol in rat tissue. J Biol Chem 250:299.

Haddad JG, Boisseau V, Avioli LV 1971 Placental transfer of vitamin D and 25-hydroxycholecalciferol in the rat. J Lab Clin Med 77:908.

Haddad JG, Walgate J 1976 Radioimmunoassay of binding protein for vitamin D and its metabolites in human serum. Concentrations in normal subjects and patients with disorders of mineral homeostasis. J Clin Invest 58:1217.

Hafez ESE 1970 Reproduction and breeding techniques for laboratory animals, Philadelphia, Lea & Febiger, pp 299.

Halloran BP, Barthell EM, De Luca HF 1979 Vitamin D metabolism during pregnancy and lactation in the rat. Proc Natl Acad Sci USA 76:5549.

Halloran BP, De Luca HF 1980 a Effect of vitamin D deficiency on fertility and reproductive capacity in female rat. J Nutr 110:1573.

Halloran BP, De Luca HF 1980 b Calcium transport in small intestine during pregnancy and lactation. Am J Physiol 239: E64.

Halloran BP, De Luca HF 1980 c Skeletal changes during pregnancy and lactation: The role of vitamin D. Endocrinology 107:1923.

Halloran BP, De Luca HF 1981 Effect of vitamin D on skeletal development during early growth in the rat. Arch Biochem Biophys 209: 7.

Harding JC, Cairnie AB 1975 Changes in intestinal cell kinetics in small intestine of lactating mice. Cell Tissue Kinet 8:135.

Hariharan S 1985 Nutrition of laboratory animals, In: Laboratory animal information service news, Hyderabad, National Institute of Nutrition. P49.

Harrison M, Fraser R 1960 Bone structure and metabolism in calcium deficient rats. J Endocrinol 21:197.

Haussler MR 1986 Vitamin D receptors: Nature and function. Ann Rev Nutr 6:527.

Haussler MR, Donaldson CA, Kelly MA et al. 1985 Functions and mechanism of action of 1,25-dihydroxyvitamin D_3 receptor, In: Vitamin D: A chemical, biochemical and clinical update, ed Norman et al. Berlin, Walter de Gruyter, pp 83.

Haussler MR, Manolagas SC, Debtos LJ 1982 Receptors for 1,25-dihydroxyvitamin D3 in GH3 pituitary cells. J steroid biochem 16:15.

Haussler MR, Myrtle JF,Norman AW. The association of a metabolite of vitamin D_3 with intestinal mucosa chromatin, in vivo. J Biol Chem 1968; 243:4055-4064.

Heaney RP, Skilman TG 1971 Calcium metabolism in normal human pregnancy. J Clin Endocrinol Metab 33:661.

Heckmatt JZ, Peacock M, Davies AE, McMurry J, Ishewood DM 1979 Plasma 25-hydroxyvitamin D in pregnant Asian women and their babies. Lancet ii:546.

Hellman P, Liu W, Westing G, Torma H, Aperstrom G1999 Vitamin D and retinoids in parathyroid glands (review). Int J Mol Med 4:355.

Henning H, Michael D, Cheng C et al. 1980 Calcium regulation of growth and differentiation of mouse epidermal cells in culture. Cell 19:245.

Henry HL, Norman AW1975 Studies on the mechanism of action of calciferol VII. Localization of 1,25-dihydroxyvitamin D3 in chick parathyroid glands. Biochem Biophys Res Commun 62:781.

Henry HL, Norman AW 1978 Vitamin D: two dihydroxylated metabolites are required for normal chicken egg hatchability. Science 201:835.

Hess AF and Weinstock M 1924 Antirachitic properties imparted to inert fluids and to green vegetables by ultraviolet irradiation. J Biol Chem 62:301.

Hibbs JW, Ponden WB 1955 Studies on milk fever in dairy cows. IV. Prevention by short-time prepartum feeding of massive doses of vitamin D. J Dairy Sci 38:65.

Hidiroglou M, Williams CJ, 1981 Transfer of tritium labeled vitamin D_3 in ovine placenta. Am J Vet Res 42:140.

Holick MF 1986 Vitamin D requirements for elderly. Clin Nutr 5:121.

Holick MF, MacLaughlin JA, Clark BM, et al. 1980 Photosynthesis of previtamin D_3 in human skin and physiologic consequences. Science 210:203.

Holick MF, MacLaughlin JA, Doppelt SH 1981 Factors that influence the cutaneous photosynthesis of previtamin D_3. Science 211: 509.

Holick MF, Potts JT, Krane SM 1986 Calcium, phosphorus and vitamin D metabolism, In: Harrison's Principles of Internal Medicine (11th Ed) Ed Braundwald E et al. New york, McGraw-Hill, pp 1857.

Holick MF, Schnoes HK, De Luca HF, Sida T, Cousine RF 1971 Isolation and identification of 1,25-dihydroxycholecalciferol, a metabolite of vitamin D active in intestine. Biochemistery 10: 2799.

Hollis BW, Hibbs JW, Conrad HR 1977 Vitamin D binding factors in bovine blood. J Dairy Sci 60:1605.

Hollis BW, Johnson D, Hulsey TC, Wbeling M, Wagner CL 2011 Vitamin D supplementation during pregnancy: double blind randomized clinical trial of safety and effectiveness. J Bone Miner Res 26: 2341.

Hollis BW, Roos BA, Draper HH, Lambert PW 1981 Vitamin D and its metabolites in human and bovine milk. J Nutr 111:240.

Holtrop ME, Cox KA, Carnes DL, Holick MF 1986 Effects of serum calcium and phosphorus on skeletal mineralization in vitamin D-deficient rats. Am J Physiol: E234.

Holtrop ME, Cox KA, Clark MB, Holick MF , Anast CS 1981 1,25-dihydroxycholecalciferol stimulates osteoclasts in rat bones in the absence of parathyroid hormone. Endocrinology 108:2293.

Holtrop ME, Holick MF, Carnes DL 1982 A vitamin D deficient rat model with normal serum calcium and serum parathyroid hormone and absence of rickets and osteomalacia. Calci Tissue Int 34: Suppl S 52.

Hosomi JJ, Hosoi E, Suda AT, Kiroki T.1978 Regulation of terminal differentiation of cultured mouse epidermal cells by 1,25 –dihydroxy vitamin D_3. Endocrinology113: 1 950.

Hove K 1981 A permanent preparation allowing measurement of secretions of parathyroid hormone in conscious goats. J Endocrinol 90:295.

Howard GA, Turner RT, Puzas JE et al. 1982 Bone cells in culture synthesize 1,25 (OH)2 D3 as determined by mass spectrometry, In Vitamin D: A chemical, biochemical and clinical update, Ed Norman et al. Berlin, Walter de Gruyter, pp 3.

Howard GA, Turner RT, Sherrard DJ, Baylink DJ 1981 Human bone cells in culture metabolize 25-hydroxyvitamin D3 to 1,25-dihydroxyvitamin D_3 and 24,25-dihydroxy vitamin D_3. J Biol Chem 256:7738.

Hughes MR, Brumbaugh PF, Haussler MR et al. 1975 Regulation of serum 1,25-dihydroxyvitamin D3 by calcium and phosphate in the rat. Science 190:578.

Imawari M, Goodman DS 1976 The transport of vitamin D and its 25-hydroxy-metabolite in human plasma. Isolation and partial characterization of vitamin D and 25-hydroxyvitamin D binding protein. J Clin Invest 58:514.

Iwasaki Y, Iwasaki J, Freake HC 1983 Growth inhibition of human breast cancer cells induced by calcitonin. Biochem Biophys Res Commun 110:235.

Jeans PC, Stearns G 1938 The effect of vitamin D on linear growth in infancy II.The effect of above 1800 USP units daily. J Pediatr 13:730.

Jones G, Strugnell SA, DeLuca HF 1998 Current understanding of the molecular action of vitamin D. Physiol Rev 78:1194.

Kent GN, Price RS, Gutteridge DH et al. 1991 The efficiency of intestinal calcium absorption is increased in late pregnancy but not in lactation. Calcif Tissue Int 48:293.

Korenchevsky V, Carr M 1923 The influence of mother's diet during pregnancy and lactation on the growth, general nourishment and skeleton of rats. J Pathol Bacteriol 26:389.

Kostial K, Durakovic A, Simonovic I, Juvancic V 1969 a The effect of some dietary additives on calcium and strontium absorption in suckling and lactating rats. Int J Pediat Biol 15:563.

Kostial K, Gruden N, Durakovic A 1969 b Intestinal absorption of calcium-47 and strontium-85 in lactating rats. Calcif Tissue Res 4:13.

Kumar R, Cohen WR Silve P, Epstein PH 1979 Elevated 1,25-dihydroxyvitamin D plasma levels in normal human pregnancy and lactation. J Clin Invest 63:342.

Kwiecinski GG, Petrie GF, DeLuca HF.1989 Vitamin D is necessary for reproductive functions in the male Rat. J Nutr. 119: 741.

Lambert PW, De Oreo PD, Hollis BW et al.1981 Concurrent measurement of plasma levels of vitamin D3 and five of its metabolites in normal, chronic renal failure and anephric humans. J Lab Clin Med 98:536.

Larson BL, Jagrensen GN 1974 Biosynthesis of milk proteins, In: Lactation :Biosynthesis and Secretion of Milk, Ed Larson BL, Smith VR New York, Academic press, pp 115.

Larson S, Biquist L 1977 Low doses of 1, 25 dihydroxycholecalciferol increase bone mass in adult normal rat. Clin Ortho Rel Res 127:228.

Laundry CS, Ruppe MD, Grubbs EG 2011 Vitamin D receptors and parathyroid glands. Endocr Pract 2011;Suppl 1:63

Lio SH, Chu HL 1943 Studies of calcium and phosphorus metabolism with special reference to pathogenesis and effects of dihydrotachysterol (AT 10). Medicine 22:103.

Liu SH, Chu HI, Su CC et al. 1940 Calcium and phosphorus metabolism in osteomalacia. IX Metabolic behavior of infants fed on breast milk from mothers showing states of vitamin D nutrition. J Clin Invest 19:327.

Liu SH, Su CC, Wang CW, Chang KP 1937 Calcium and phosphorus metabolism in osteomalacia.VI The added drain of lactation and beneficial actions of vitamin D. Chin J Physiol 11:271.

Lo CW, Paris PW, Clemens TL et al. 1985 Vitamin D absorption in healthy subjects and in patients with intestinal malabsorption syndrome. Am J Clin Nutr 42:644.

Long RG, Skinner RK, Meinhard E et al. 1976 Serum 25-hydroxyvitaminD values in liver disease and hepatic osteomalacia. Gut 17:824.

Loomis WF 1967 Skin-pigment regulation of vitamin D biosynthesis in man. Science 157:501.

Lund B, Selnes A 1979 Plasma 1,25-dihydroxyvitamin D levels in pregnancy and lactation. Acta Endocrinol 92:330.

MacLaughlin JA, Anderson RR, Holoick MR 1982 Special character of sunlight modulates the photosynthesis of provitamin D3 and its photoisomers in human skin. Science 216: 1001.

MacLaughlin JA, Holick MF 1985 Aging decreases the capacity of human skin to produce vitamin D_3. J Clin Invest 76: 1536.

MacLennan WJ, Hamilton JC, Darmady JM 1980 The effect of season and stage of pregnancy on plasma 25-hydroxyvitamin D concentrations in pregnant women. Postgrad Med J 56: 75.

Mainoya JR 1975 a Effect of bovine growth hormone, human placental lactogen and ovine prolactin on intestinal fluid and ion transport in the rat. Endocrinology 96: 1165.

Mainoya JR 1975 b Further studies on the action of prolactin on fluid and ion absorption by rat jejunum. Endocrinology 96: 1158.

Mainoya JR 1978 Possible influence of prolactin on intestinal hypertrophy in pregnant and lactating rat. Experientia 34:1230.

Marya RK, Rathee S, Dua V,Sangwan K 1988 Effect of vitamin D supplementation during pregnancy on fetal growth. Ind J Med Res 88:448

Marya RK, Rathee S, Lata V, Mudgil S.1981a Effects of vitamin D supplementation in pregnancy. Gynaecol Obstet Invest 12:155.

Marya RK, Saini AS, Rathee S, Arora SR. 1981 b Osteomalacia in Hindu population of Haryana. Ind J Med Res 73:756.

Mathian CJ, Laureys J, Sobis H, Vandeputtle MV, Boillon R 1992 1,25-dihydroxyvitamin D_3 prevents insulitis in NOD mice. Diabetes 41:1491

Matsuoko L, Wortsman J, MacLaughlin JA, Holick MF 1987 Sunscreen suppresses cutaneous vitamin D_3 synthesis. J Clin Endocrinol Metab 64:1165.

Maxwell JD, Aug L, Brooke OG, Brown IRF 1981 Vitamin D supplements enhance weight gain and nutritional status in pregnant Asians. Br J Obstet Gynaecol 88:987.

Maxwell JP, Miles LM 1925 Osteomalacia in China. J Obstet Gynaecol Br Emp 32:433.

Maxwell JP, Pi HT, Lin HAC, Kue CC 1939 Further studies in adult rickets (osteomalacia) and foetal rickets. Proc Soc Med 32:287.

Mayer E, Kadowaski S, Williams G, Norman AW.1984 Mode of action of 1,25-dihydroxyvitamin D, In: Vitamin D: Basic and Clinical Aspects, Ed Kumar R, Boston, Martinus Nijhoff, pp 259.

McCollem EW, Simonds N, Becker JE, Shipley PG 1925 Studies on experimental rickets XXVI. A diet composed principally of purified foodstuffs for use with 'line test' for vitamin D studies. J Biol Chem 65:97

Mellenby E 1918 a The part played by accessory food factor in the production of experimental rickets. J Physiol (Lond) 52:XI.

Mellenby E 1918 b A further demonstration of the part played by accessory food factors in the aetiology of rickets. J Physiol (Lond) 52: LIII.

Mellenby E 1919 An experimental investigation in rickets. Lancet 97:407.

Mendelsohn M, Haddad JG, 1975 Postnatal fall and rise of circulating 1,25-dihydroxyvitamin D in the rat. J Lab Clin Med 86: 32.

Miller SC, Halloran BP, De Luca HF, Jee WSS 1982 The role of vitamin D in maternal skeletal changes during pregnancy and lactation. A histomorpho-metric study. Calcif Tissue Intl 34:245.

Morimoto S, Onishi T, Imanaka S, et al. 1986 Administration of 1,25-dihydroxyvitamin D3 for psoriasis: report of five cases. Calcif Tissue Intl 38: 119.

Naismith DJ 1966 The requirement for protein and utilization of protein and calcium during pregnancy. Metabolism 15:582.

Nakamura T, Kurokova T, Oromo H 1988 Increase of bone volume in vitamin D-repleted rats by massive administration of 24,25 $(OH)_2$ D_3. Calcif Tissue Int 43:235.

Narbiatz R, Sar M, Stumpf WE et al. 1981 1, 25-dihydroxyvitamin D_3 targets cells in rat mammary gland. Horm Res 15: 263.

Oh YJ, Horst RL 1981 Vitamin D metabolites in colostrum and milk from normal, vitamin D3 and 1,25-dihydroxyvitamin D3-treated cows. Fed Proc 40: 895.

Olson EB, De Luca HF 1973 Vitamin D metabolism and mechanism of action. World Rev Nutr Dietet 17: 104.

Olson EB, Knutson JC, Bhattacharya MH, De Luca HF 1976 The effect of hepatectomy on synthesis of 25-hydroxyvitamin D3. J Clin Invest 57:1213.

Parez R, Raab TC, Turner CA, Holick MF 1996 Safety and efficacy of oral calciferol (1,25-dihydroxyvitamin D_3) for the treatment of psoriasis. Br J Dermatol 134:1070.

Patterson AM 1952 Nomenclature. Words about words. Chem Eng News 30: 104.

Paunier L, Lacourt G, Pilloud P et al. 1978 25-hydroxyvitamin D and calcium levels in maternal, cord and infant serum in relation to maternal vitamin D intake. Helv Paediatr Acta 33: 95.

Phuja DN, De Luca HF 1981 Stimulationn of intestinal calcium transport and bone calcium mobilization in vitamin D-deficient rats. Science 214:1038.

Pietrek J, Kokot F. 1977 Serum 25-hydroxyvitamin D in patients with chronic renal disease. Eur J Clin Invest 7: 282.

Pike JW, Parker JB, Haussler MR et al. 1979 Dynamic changes in circulating 1,25-dihydroxyvitamin D during reproduction in rats. Science 204: 1427.

Pitkin RM, Reynolds WA, Williams CA 1979 Calcium metabolism in pregnancy: a longitudinal study. Am J Obstet Gynecol 53: 746.

Polskin J, Kramer B, Sobel AE 1945 Secretion of vitamin D in milks of women fed fish liver oil. J Nutr 30: 451.

Ponchon G, De Luca HF 1969 The role of liver in the metabolism of vitamin D. J Clin Invest 77: 7.

Portale AA, Halloran BP, Murphy MM, Morris RC 1986 Oral intake of phosphorus can determine the serum concentration of 1,25-dihydroxyvitamin D by determining its production rate in humans. J Clin Invest 77: 7.

Porter G 1963 Feeding rats and mice, In: Animals for research, Ed Lane-Petter W, London, Academic press, pp 27.

Price PA 1984 The effect of 1, 25-dihysroxyvitamin D_3 on synthesis of vitamin K-dependent protein of bone, In: Vitamin D: Basic and Clinical Aspects, Ed Kumar R, Boston, Martinus Nijhoff, pp 397.

Provvedini DM, Rulot CM, Sobal RE, Tsoukas, CD, Manolagas SC 1987 1, 25-Dihydroxyvitamin D_3 receptors in human thymic and tonsillar lymphocytes. J Bone Miner Res 2: 239

Provvdine DM, Tsoukas CD, Deftos LJ, Manolagas SC 1983 1, 25-dihydroxyvitamin D3 receptors in human leucocytes. Science 221:1181.

Puri M, Rathee S, Marya, RK. 1989 Calcium and vitamin D supplements in pregnant women: effect on fetal weight. J Obstet Gynecol India. 39,307.

Rasmussen P 1969 Action of vitamin D deficiency on bone tissues and epiphyseal plate in rats given adequate amounts of calcium and phosphorus in the diet. Arch Oral biol 14: 1293.

Rasmussen P 1977 a Calcium deficiency, pregnancy, and lactation in rats. Some effects on blood chemistry and the skeleton. Calcif Tissue Res 23: 87.

Rasmussen P 1977 b Calcium deficiency, pregnancy, and lactation in rats. Microscopic and microradiographic observations in bones. Calcif Tissue Res 23: 95.

Reichel H, Koeffler HP, Normen A 1989 The role of vitamin D endocrine system in health and disease. N Engl J Med 320: 980.

Reinhardt TA, Conrad HR 1980 Specific binding protein for 1, 25-dihydroxyvitamin D_3 in bovine mammary tissue. Arch Biochem Biophys 203: 108.

Reitz RE, Daane TA, Woods JR, Weinstein RL 1977 Calcium, magnesium, phosphorus and parathyroid hormone interrelationships in pregnancy and new born infants. Obstet Gynecol 50: 701.

Retallack RW, Jeffroes M, Kent GN et al. 1977 Physiological hyperparathyroidism in human lactation. Calcif Tissue Res 22 (Suppl): 142.

Rosen JF, Roginsky M, Mathensen G, Finberg L 1974 25-hydroxyvitamin D: Plasma levels in mothers and their premature infants with neonatal hypocalcemia. Am J Dis Child 127:220.

Rosenheim O, Webster TA 1925 Rickets and cholesterol. Lancet i: 1025.

Rosenthal N, Insonga KL, Godsall JW et al. 1985 Elevations in 1,25-dihydroxyvitamin D3 in patients with lymphoma-associated hypercalcemia. J Clin Endocrinol Metab 60: 29.

Ross R, Care AD, Taylor CM et al. 1979 The transplacental transfer of metabolites of vitamin D in sheep, In: Vitamin D: Chemical, Biochemical and Clinical Update. Ed Norman et al. Walter de Gruyter, pp 241.

Rosso P 1977 Effects of maternal dietary restrictions during pregnancy on fetal growth and maternal-fetal exchange in mammalian species, In: Nutritional Impacts on women, Ed Moghissi KS, Evans TN, New York, Harper & Row, pp 56.

Sachan A, Gupta R, Das V, Aggarwal A 2005 High prevalence of vitamin D deficiency amonst pregnant women and newborns in northern India. Am J Clin Nutr 81:1060

Sar M, Stumb WE, DE Luca HF 1980 Thyrotropes in pituitary are target cells for 1,25-dihydroxyvitamin D_3. Cell Tissue Res 209: 161.

Schedwie H, Slikker W, Hill D et al. 1980 Placental crossover and fetal tissue distribution of 1,25(OH)2 vitamin D in rhesus monkey. Pediatr Res 14: 58.

Schneider WC 1957 Determination of nucleic acids in tissues by pentose analysis. Meth Enzymol 3: 680.

Shepard RM, Horst RL, Hamstra AJ, DE Luca HF 1979 Determination of vitamin D and its metabolites in plasma from normal and anephric man. Biochem J 182:55.

Shohl AT 1936 Rickets in rats. The effect of low calcium-high phosphorus diet in various levels and ratios upon the production of rickets and tetany. J Nutr 11: 275.

Sergio A, Lipkin L, Lipkin M 2003 Chemoprevention of colon cancer by calcium, vitamin D and folate. Nature Rev Cancer 2003; 3:601

Slyker F, Hamil EM, Poole MW et al. 1937 Relationship between vitamin D intake and linear growth in infants. Proc Soc Exper Biol Med 37: 499.

Smith JJ, Park CS, Keenon TW 1982 Calcium and calcium inophore A23187 alter protein synthesis and secretion by acini from rat mammary gland. Int J Biochem 14: 573.

Smith EL, Walworth NC, Holick MF 1986 Effect of 1,25-dihydroxyvitamin D3 on morphologic and biochemical differentiation of cultured human epidermal keratinocytes growth in serum-free conditions. J Invest Dermatol 86: 709.

Snapper I 1956 Osteomalacia in North China; Its relationship to pregnancy and lactation.Ann N Y Acad Sci 86: 709.

Sood S, Marya RK, Reghunandanan R, Singh GP, Jaswal TS, Gopinathan K 1992 Effect of vitamin D deficiency on testicular function in the rat. Ann Nutr Metab 36:203

Sood S, Reghunandanan R, Reghunandanan V, Marya RK, Singh PI.1995 Effect of vitamin D repletion on testicular function in vitamin D-deficient rats. Ann Nutr Metab 39:95

Spanos E, Berrett D, MacIyntyr I et al. 1976 Effect of growth hormone on vitamin D metabolism. Nature 273: 246

Spanos E, Coloston KW, Evans IMS et al. 1976 Effect of prolactin on vitamin D metabolism. Mol Cell Endocrinol 5: 163.

Spray CM 1950 A study of some aspects of reproduction by means of chemical analysis. Br J Nutr 4: 354.

Stearns G, Jeans PC, Vandecar V 1936 Effect of vitamin d on linear growth in infancy. J Pediatr 9: 1.

Steenbock H 1924 The induction of growth promoting and calcifying properties in a ration by exposure to light. Science 60: 224.

Steenbock H, Black A 1925 Fat soluble vitamins XXIII. The induction of growth promoting and calcifying properties in fats and their unsaponifiable constituents by exposure to light. J Biol Chem 64: 263.

Steenbock H, Herting DC 1955 Vitamin D and growth. J Nutr 57:449.

Steichen JJ, Tsang RC, Gratton TL 1980 Vitamin D homeostasis in the perinatal period: 1,25-dihydroxyvitamin D in maternal, cord and neonatal blood. N Engl J Med 302: 315.

Stewart RJC 1975 Bone pathology in experimental rickets. World Rev Nutr 21: 1.

Stumpf WE, Sar M, Reid FA et al. 1979 Target cells for 1,25-dihydroxyvitamin D3 in intestinal tract, stomach, kidney, skin, pituitary and parathyroid. Science 206: 1188.

Suda T, Kurokowa K 1983 Characteristic localization of 25-hydroxyvitamin D3 hydroxylase along fetal nephron, In: Perinatal calcium and phosphorus metabolism. Ed Holick MF, Gray TK, Anast CS, Amsterdam, Elsevier. pp 57.

Sunde ML, Turk CM, De Luca HF 1978 The essentiality of vitamin D metabolites for embryonic development. Science 200: 1067.

Tanaka Y, Castillo L, De Luca HF 1976 Control of renal vitamin D hydroxylases in birds by sex hormones. Proc Natl Acad Sci USA 73: 2701.

Tanaka Y, Castillo L, Wineland MJ, De Luca HF 1978 Synergistic effect of progesterone, testosterone, and estradiol in stimulation of chick renal 25-hydroxyvitamin D3-hydroxylase. Endocrinology 103: 2035.

Toverud SU, Boass A 1979 Hormonal control of calcium metabolism in lactation. Vitam Horm 37:303.

Toverud SU, Boass A, Munson PL 1978 Elevated intestinal calcium absorption in vitamin D-deprived lactating rats. US Endocr Soc Abstr No 318, p 233.

Toverud SU, Harper C, Munson PL 1976 Calcium metabolism during lactation: enhanced effect of thyrocalcitonin. Endocrinology 99: 371.

Tucker G, Gagnon RE, Haussler MR 1973 Vitamin D3-25 hydroxylase: Tissue occurrence and apparent lack of regulation. Arch Biochem Biophys 155: 47.

Turner RT, Puzas JE, Forte MD, Baylink DJ 1980 Production of 1,25 (OH)2 D3 by cultured embryonic chick calvarias cells. Proc Natl Acad Sci USA 77: 5750.

Turton CWG, Stanley P, Stamp TCB, Maxwell JD 1977 Altered vitamin D metabolism in pregnancy. Lancet 1: 222.

Twardock AR, Austin MK 1970 Calcium transfer in perfused guinea pig placenta. Am J Physiol 219: 540.

Vanbaelen H, Bouillon R, DeMoor P 1977 Binding of 25-hydroxychole-calciferol in tissues. J Biol Chem 252: 2515.

Wasserman RH, Fullmer CS, Shimura F 1984 Calcium absorption and the molecular effects of vitamin D3, In: Vitamin D: Basic and Clinical Aspects, Ed Kumar R, Boston, Martinus Nijhoff, pp 233.

Watney PJM, Rudd BT 1974 Calcium metabolism in pregnancy and in the new born. J Obstet Gynaecol Br Commn 81: 210.

Webb AR, deCosta B, Holick MF 1986 Effect of winter solar irradiation on photochemistry of 7-dehydrocholesterol, its photoisomers and vitamin D3. Photochem Photobiol 43s: 1165.

Weisman Y, Occhipinti M, Knox G et al. 1978 a Concentrations of 24, 25- dihydroxyvitamin D and 25-hydroxyvitamin D in paired maternal-cord sera. Am J Obstet Gynecol 130: 704.

Weisman Y, Sapir R, Harrel A, EdelsteinS 1976 Maternal perinatal interrelationship of vitamin D in rats. Biochem Biophys Acta 428:388.

Weisman Y, Vargas A, Duckett G et al. 1978 b Synthesis of 1, 25-dihydroxyvitamin D in nephrectomised pregnant rat. Endocrinology 103: 1992.

Whitehead M, Lana G, Young O et al. 1981 Interrelationship of calcium-regulating hormones during normal pregnancy. Br Med J 282:10.

Whitfield JF, Boynton Al, MacManus JP et al. 1980 The roles of calcium and cyclic AMP in cell proliferation. Ann NY Acad Sci 339: 216.

Whitsett JA, Ho M, Tsang RC et al. 1981 Synthesis of 1,25-dihydroxyvitamin D3 by human placenta in vitro. J Clin Endocrinol Metab 53: 484.

Widdowson EM, Crabb DE, Milner RDG 1972 Cellular development of some human organs before birth. Arch Dis Childh 47: 652.

Wieland P, Fischer JA, Trechsel U et al. 1980 Perinatal parathyroid hormone, vitamin D metabolites and calcitonin in man. Am J Physiol 239: E 385.

Winick M, Brasel JA, Rasso P 1972 Nutrition and cell growth, In:Current Concepts in Nutrition, ed Winick M, New York, John Willey, pp 15.

Winick M, Noble A 1965 Quantitative changes in DNA, RNA and protein during prenatal and postnatal growth in the rat. Dev Biol 12:451.

Winick M, Noble A 1967 Cellular response with increased feeding in neonatal rat. J Nutr 91: 179.

Work JD, Tashjian AH 1982 Vitamin D stimulates prolactin synthesis by GH_4C_1 cells incubated in chemically defined medium. Endocrinology 111: 1755.

Work JD, Tashjian AH 1982 Vitamin D stimulates prolactin synthesis by GH_4C_1 cells incubated in chemically defined medium. Endocrinology 111: 1755.

Yang SC, Smith JM, Prahl JM, DeLuca HF 1983 Vitamin D deficiency suppresses cell mediated immunity in vivo. Arch Biochem Biophys 303:98

Zaloga GP, Eli C, Medberg CA 1985 Humoral hypercalcemia in Hidgkin's disease, Arch Intern Med 145: 155.

Zerwelh JW, Sakhee K, Pak CYC 1985 Short term 1,25-dihydroxyvitamin D3 raises serim osteocalcin in patients with postmenopausal osteoporosis. J Clin Endocrinol Metab 60: 615.

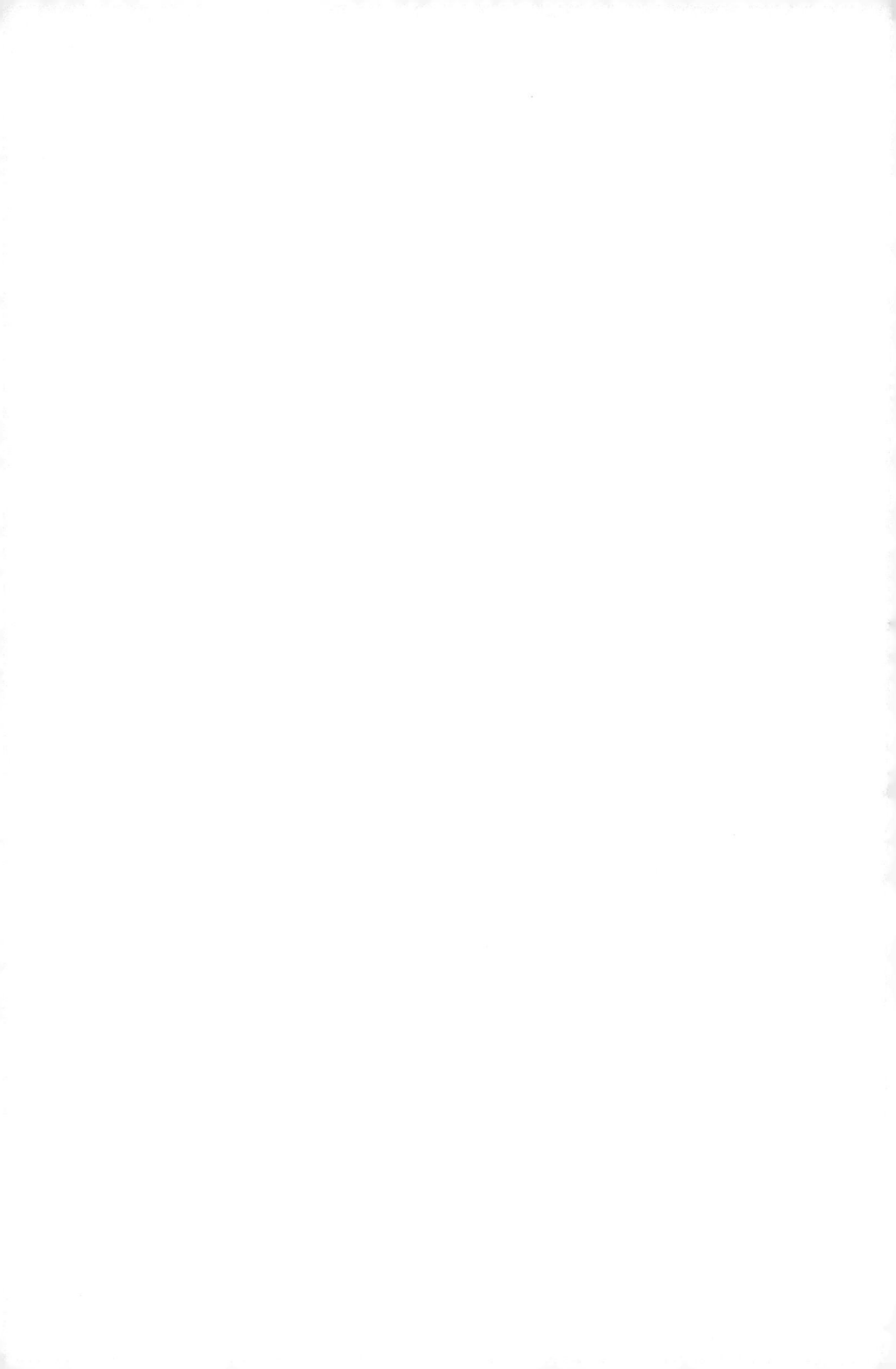